Medical Aspects of Anorexia Nervosa

Medical Aspects of Anorexia Nervosa

S BHANJI MD (Lond), FRCPsych
Senior Lecturer in Adult Mental Illness,
Postgraduate Medical School, University of Exeter;
Consultant Psychiatrist, Exeter Health Authority

D MATTINGLY MB, FRCP(Lond)
Emeritus Professor of Postgraduate Medical Studies and
formerly Director, Postgraduate Medical School,
University of Exeter;
Honorary Consultant Physician, Royal Devon and Exeter
Hospital.

Wright
London   Boston   Singapore   Sydney   Toronto   Wellington

Wright
is an imprint of Butterworth Scientific

All rights reserved. No part of this publication may be reproduced or transmitted in any form or by any means, including photocopying and recording, without the written permission of the copyright holder, application for which should be addressed to the Publishers, or in accordance with the provisions of the Copyright Act 1956 (as amended), or under the terms of any licence permitting limited copying issued by the Copyright Licensing Agency, 7 Ridgemount Street, London WC1E 7AE, England. Such written permission must also be obtained before any part of this publication is stored in a retrieval system of any nature.

Any person who does any unauthorized act in relation to this publication may be liable to criminal prosecution and civil claims for damages.

This book is sold subject to the Standard Conditions of Sale of Net Books and may not re-sold in the UK below the net price given by the Publishers in their current price list.

First published, 1988

© **Butterworth & Co. (Publishers) Ltd, 1988**

British Library Cataloguing in Publication Data

Bhanji, S.
 Medical aspects of anorexia nervosa.
 1. Man. Anorexia nervosa
 I. Title II. Mattingly, D.
 616.85′2

ISBN 0–7236–1115 7

Library of Congress Cataloging in Publication Data

Bhanji, S.
 Medical aspects of anorexia nervosa.

 Includes bibliographies and index.
  I. Anorexia nervosa—Physiological aspects.
 2. Anorexia nervosa—Complications and sequelae.
 I. Mattingly, David. II. Title. [DNLM: 1. Anorexia Nervosa. WM 175 B575m]
 RC552.A5B48 1988   616.85′2   88–267
 ISBN 0–7236–1115 7

Typeset by Latimer Trend & Company Ltd, Plymouth
Printed and bound in Great Britain by Anchor Brendon Ltd, Tiptree, Essex

Preface

Anorexia nervosa is a potentially fatal disorder primarily affecting adolescent girls and young women and appears to be becoming more prevalent. The true nature of the condition is still unknown in spite of accounts dating from over three centuries ago and the recent attention paid to it by the media. It has been variously described as a psychiatric disorder, an endocrine and metabolic disturbance, or a combination of both.

This book was written in an attempt to focus on those medical aspects of anorexia nervosa which may affect both management and prognosis, and to discuss its treatment. We have drawn upon our own experience of 155 cases seen in a District General Hospital over the last 20 years. Many of the earlier accounts of this disorder were written by physicians, but in more recent years the majority of publications have concentrated on the psychiatric, psychological, and sociological aspects. Nevertheless, the investigation and management of the anorectic are by no means the exclusive province of the psychiatrist. It is probable that at least half of the anorectics seen in the UK are still treated at some stage of the illness by physicians.

In the UK the prevalence of anorexia nervosa among those at greatest risk, namely white middle-class adolescent girls, is of the order of 1%. Estimates of mortality vary enormously. Some follow-up studies have revealed no fatalities, but in one series almost one-quarter had died. The average mortality rate would appear to be of the order of 5–10%, death resulting from gross electrolyte depletion, infection, complications of treatment, or suicide. Anorexia nervosa is also responsible for much morbidity and the physical complications of this disease often pass unrecognized.

Bulimia nervosa, which is also an eating disorder, is discussed only briefly. Its complications are similar to those which may be found in anorectics who periodically binge and indulge in self-induced vomiting or laxative and diuretic abuse. There is as yet no agreement as to whether bulimia nervosa is a variant of anorexia nervosa or a separate condition.

S. Bhanji
D. Mattingly

Acknowledgements

Our interest in anorexia nervosa could not have flourished without the goodwill and expertise of many of our colleagues at the University of Exeter Postgraduate Medical School and the Royal Devon and Exeter Hospital. We are particularly indebted to Sister Lyn Taylor and her nurses, and the numerous junior medical staff who collaborated in the investigation and treatment of our anorectics on Torridge Ward. Special gratitude is owed to Dr T. Hargreaves and Mr J. Barraclough for carrying out the biochemical and endocrinological investigations, and to Dr Josephine Arendt and Christine Franey of the Department of Biochemistry of the University of Surrey for estimating plasma melatonin concentrations. The last could not have been carried out without a generous grant from the Northcott Devon Medical Foundation. The cooperation of Drs C. R. B. Bayliss and M. D. McLean proved invaluable in our studies of the radiological changes, and Professor P. P. Anthony willingly traced and re-examined histological material from a previous study. Mrs Alison Murray drew our attention to a nutritional knowledge questionnaire and advised over its use.

Thanks are also due to Dr Valerie Jones, Dr Christine Tyler, Dr David Shaw, Mr James Ladd and Mrs Amanda Hesford for their helpful comments and suggestions regarding various chapters.

The figures were prepared by Mr Harold Martin, and Mr T. Gooch and his colleagues. The manuscript was typed by Mrs Mary Wood. Without the latter's dedication and skill this book would have still been in preparation.

Contents

Preface		v
Acknowledgements		vii
1	Historical background	1
2	Aetiology	7
3	Clinical features	15
4	The authors' series	22
5	The cardiovascular system	27
6	The respiratory system	34
7	The nervous system	37
8	The alimentary tract	46
9	Haematology and immunology	55
10	Renal function and electrolytes	63
11	The endocrine system	71
12	Cholesterol and carotene	86
13	Nutritional disorders	92
14	Psychiatric management	100
15	Medical management	105
16	The authors' management regimen	113
17	Prognosis	121
18	Bulimia nervosa	127
Appendix: Normal values		133
Index		135

Chapter 1

Historical background

Early fasters

The first account of a disorder recognizable as anorexia nervosa appeared towards the end of the seventeenth century (Morton, 1689), and earlier literature contains many reports of people who starved themselves deliberately. Some of these, and various historical figures such as Richard II (Yearsley, 1935) and Mary, Queen of Scots (McSherry, 1985) may have been suffering from this disease. Hammond (1879) and Gould and Pyle (1901) mention many early medieval records of those claiming divine or satanic assistance in existing on little or no nourishment. They were followed in later centuries by the 'miraculous fasters', usually adolescent girls, who, following illness or injury, lost all inclination to eat or drink. These girls attracted considerable local and national attention, and frequently received distinguished visitors who were expected to leave behind a gift.

An early example is Jane Balan (Mexio, 1613; Morgan, 1977), the 14-year-old daughter of a French locksmith who was said to have lived for 3 years without food or drink; reportedly during that time no urine or faeces were passed and no menstruation occurred. Her history began with a fever which commenced on 16 February 1599, accompanied by vomiting, and which lasted some 3 weeks. Jane was then mute for a month and when her speech did return she was delirious. She was also paralysed and no-one could persuade her to eat. Some 6 months later she regained her strength and wits, although her reluctance to eat persisted. Her abdomen became wasted as if all its viscera had been removed. By contrast the limbs, face and breasts were quite fleshy.

Two later cases attracted widespread attention and concern. Sarah Jacob, 'the Welsh fasting girl', was born in May 1857 to parents described as uneducated, ignorant and simple-minded farmers (Hammond, 1879; Morgan, 1977). One day in February 1867 she complained of abdominal pain and told her mother that on waking her mouth was full of blood and froth. The pain continued and soon Sarah developed convulsions and muscle spasms. Some writers have regarded the last as opisthotonos and others as a sign of hysteria. After a period of unconsciousness during which it was thought she was dying, she began to recover. Sarah was, however, unable to eat or drink and according to herself and her family ceased to take any nourishment from 10 October 1867. She soon became the subject of much interest and was visited by the local vicar. Although at first sceptical he became convinced that her story was true, and published a letter disputing the medical view that Sarah was no more than a fraud. This led to a local committee being appointed to observe the girl constantly for a period of 2 weeks. Their task, however, was poorly regulated and conducted.

Only the parents had free access to Sarah's bed. Some of the watchers were biased, some were unpunctual, and some were drunk. In August 1869 Sarah was visited by a Dr Fowler, who wrote a letter to *The Times* which renewed public interest and led to a second and more stringent period of observation by four nurses from Guy's Hospital, under medical supervision and with sensible precautions to avoid deception. This began on 9 December, but Sarah soon became ill and a week later the nurses urged the parents to end the experiment. They refused, even when told that Sarah was dying. In the middle of the afternoon of 16 December 1869, Sarah passed away. Public opinion was greatly aroused against those responsible, and the parents were sentenced to hard labour.

In October 1878 the *New York Herald* reported that a Miss Mary (Mollie) Fancher of Brooklyn had not eaten for 14 years (Hammond, 1879). Mollie, the child of wealthy parents, grew up as a pretty and cultured girl with all to live for. One day in 1864 she slipped while getting off a street-car. Her skirt caught on the step and Mollie was dragged some yards before the conductor realized and stopped the car. Mollie was carried home barely conscious and apparently in much pain. Two days later muscle spasms occurred and she went into a trance, being considered moribund in a similar way to Sarah Jacob. On recovery Mollie was found to be blind, to have no appetite, and to be unable to swallow. A number of doctors were interviewed regarding her anorexia and ability to see without sight. Most agreed with her story, but the regular medical attendant admitted in the end to some doubts and said he had gone along with his patient in order to establish a working relationship. Hammond suggested that the matter be put to the test, but perhaps because of his justifiable criticisms of the manner in which Sarah Jacob had been treated, did not press the issue. Nevertheless, he did throw down a challenge regarding Mollie's clairvoyance.

Whether the above patients and others like them were really suffering from anorexia nervosa is open to doubt. Even if they were not they are still important. As Morgan (1977) has pointed out, they have contributed to an attitude of mistrust and rejection among the medical profession toward young girls who starve themselves. As recently as 1979 it was stated that those suffering from anorexia nervosa are no more than deceivers and cheats, and undeserving of doctors' time and effort (Naish, 1979).

Morton's cases

Morton's account of 'nervous consumption' appeared first in Latin in 1689, with an English version in 1694. Richard Morton's life and times have been well reported by Silverman (1983), and a commentary on his treatise has been provided by Bhanji and Newton (1985). Morton described two patients, Miss Duke and Master Steele, who both developed their illness at what is now regarded as the characteristic time of life for anorexia nervosa. As with most of their modern counterparts they were born into middle-class families. Morton regarded nervous consumption as due to emotional turmoil and stressed the role of excessive educational studies in its cause. However, he based his diagnosis not on this but, as did Gull some two centuries later, on the exclusion of other known causes of wasting.

Miss Duke developed amenorrhoea and began to lose weight as a result of loss of appetite in July 1684, but did not seek Morton's help until some 3 years later after she had been troubled by fainting attacks. He described her appearance as 'like a skeleton only clad with skin', noting that her body felt cold and marvelled at Miss Duke's capacity for exercise. At first she responded to various medicines to stimulate the appetite and calm a troubled mind, but later decided to let nature take its course and died. Master Steele fared better; the turning point in his recovery may well have been Morton's advice that he give up his studies and leave home for the country.

Gull's cases

Although Morton was highly thought of and his works widely read, there was little interest in nervous consumption until the condition was rediscovered and renamed in the nineteenth century by Lasegue, in France, and Sir William Gull in England. Lasegue (1873) was the first to provide a detailed description, but precedence is usually accorded to Gull as he made a passing reference to the disease in his address to the British Medical Association in 1868. He later called the illness anorexia nervosa and presented the histories of two cases to the Clinical Society of London (Gull, 1873). From the discussion which followed it appears that many of the audience had experience of similar patients. In the following year detailed accounts of both cases and a further one were published (Gull, 1874).

Miss A, aged 17 years, first saw Gull in January 1866. She was five feet and five inches (165 cm) tall but weighed only 82 lb (37 kg) having lost some 33 lb (15 kg). Amenorrhoea had been present for one year. Although usually without appetite, there were occasions when Miss A would eat voraciously for a day or two. Gull commented on her peevish and jealous nature, and the fact that she was restless and active in spite of her emaciation. He found no internal disease, but did observe a bradycardia of 56 beats/minute. Although his early efforts were disappointing Gull persevered, and 2 years later she weighed 128 lb (58 kg) and thereafter remained in good health.

Miss B, who was 18 years old and greatly emaciated, was referred to Gull in October 1868 as a case of latent tuberculosis. Her weight was not mentioned but it was stated that no menstruation had occurred since December 1866. As with Miss A, Gull emphasized her energetic behaviour, found no sign of systemic disease, and noted a slow pulse rate. The mainstays of her treatment were 'so-called tonics' and a nourishing diet, to which she responded well.

The third case was that of Miss C, who was 15 years old when she first saw Gull in 1873. She had been ill for a year, lost much weight, and had never menstruated. Gull described her as obstinate, restless and weak-minded. Warm clothes, nourishing foods and a little brandy were prescribed, to which she seems to have responded.

Like Morton, Gull believed that anorexia nervosa derived from an abnormal state of mind. He also realized that the medication available to him was of little use. Gull advocated firm moral control, adding that the inclination of the patient must in no way be consulted; if possible she should be nursed away from family and friends. He was aware that hypothermia could occur and in such instances recommended that a rubber tube filled with warm water be placed along the spine. Gull regarded the prognosis as generally good, although he mentioned one fatal case. He was gracious enough to acknowledge the paper by Lasegue, but stressed that he had only recently been informed of it. The presence of two independent accounts strengthened his view that anorexia nervosa was a distinct condition.

Lasegue's cases

Lasegue published his account of 'l'anorexie hysterique' in 1873. An English translation appeared the same year and has recently been reprinted (Kaufman and Heiman, 1964). He based his work on eight females aged between 18 and 32 years. They all had reduced appetites and held the conviction that eating would harm them. The condition was described as having four phases. The first is ushered in by an emotionally stressful event; the patient then develops hysterical postprandial pain or discomfort and avoids food in order to feel more comfortable. Lasegue stated that this could continue for months without any significant wasting or harm to the general health. In the second phase the family becomes anxious and imploring, which serves only to consolidate the food refusal. Confident that she is doing the correct thing the girl no longer argues her case. Lasegue regarded such statements as 'je ne souffre pas donc, je suis bien portante' (I feel well, and so must be well) as virtually diagnostic. Then the illness begins to take its toll, beginning the third phase when the patient becomes aware of the family's distress and she is shocked out of her self-satisfied indifference. She is now willing to submit to treatment with enthusiasm rather than condescension. Two possible outcomes in the final phase were mentioned by Lasegue: the girl might become unconditionally obedient, but more commonly she would do just enough to avert the peril she was in without giving up her beliefs or the attention they inspired.

Like Morton and Gull, Lasegue believed that anorexia nervosa had a psychological cause. However, whereas Gull only hinted at the importance of the family, Lasegue discussed this at some length. He did not say that the family produced the illness, but was concerned that they could perpetuate it. In treating the disorder he relied heavily on persuasion, but did not favour early intervention. Instead he recommended that the doctor should remain in the background until the patient was ready to welcome him. Lasegue regarded the prognosis as good, never having seen a fatal case.

By the end of the nineteenth century anorexia nervosa was mentioned in many of the major textbooks written in English or French, but not in those in other languages. As a result it went largely unrecognized in many countries.

Twentieth century confusion

In 1914, the German pathologist, Simmonds, reported the first of a series of patients who showed no post-mortem pathology other than lesions of the pituitary gland. Some of these were emaciated. This, as Sheldon (1939) pointed out, had two regrettable consequences. The first was that any young girl who was wasting away for no obvious reason and consulted a physician who had not heard of anorexia nervosa, was likely to be incorrectly diagnosed and treated as a case of pituitary insufficiency. The second was that if the doctor realized that the symptoms were not typical, she was at risk of being regarded as having some newly discovered disease. The terms coined for this included primary atrophy of the gastric mucous membrane, asthenia gravis hypophyseogenea and wasting of late female puberty. Eventually it was shown that wasting was not a common feature of hypopituitarism and that this condition could be clearly distinguished from anorexia nervosa (Bruckner, Weis and Lavietes, 1938; Escamilla and Lisser, 1942; Sheehan and Summers, 1949). Thus, those such as Berkman (1930) in America and Ryle (1936) in England who had continued to make the diagnosis of anorexia nervosa were vindicated.

Up to the early 1940s the bulk of the literature on anorexia nervosa had come from those with an interest in internal medicine. The psychiatrists then came into the picture and brought their customary diversity of opinion. One result was that the nosological status of anorexia nervosa was again challenged. Kay and Leigh (1954), for example, investigated 38 patients diagnosed as having anorexia nervosa and concluded that they were not dealing with a specific entity. A similar but more extreme view was that adopted by Bliss and Branch (1960) whose sole diagnostic criterion was a loss of weight of 25 lb (11.4 kg) or more due to psychological causes. Other psychiatrists regarded anorexia nervosa as an unusual variant of certain specific neurotic or psychotic illnesses.

Eventually, the opinion that anorexia nervosa was a separate disorder with its characteristic clinical features and natural history, reasserted itself (Nemiah, 1958; Bruch, 1962). It now became possible to consider its classification. The division into primary and secondary types has a long history and has taken a variety of forms. Most modern writers, however, use a system similar to those propounded by King (1963) and Bruch (1966). In the primary type, the prime intent is loss of weight and the clinical features are the classical ones described by Morton, Gull and Lasegue. In secondary anorexia nervosa, the loss of weight is the result of other psychiatric illness. An example is the paranoid schizophrenic who will not eat certain food as he believes it to be poisoned.

Another widely used classification is that based on the means by which the patient reduces her net calorie intake. Meyer (1961) was the first to suggest that there are significant differences between anorectics who merely diet, and those who eat and then rid themselves of food by vomiting. Beumont, George and Smart (1976) carried out a study on 31 anorectics, 17 of whom achieved weight loss by dieting. The remaining 14 patients employed self-induced vomiting, purgatives, or diuretics as well. A number of differences were demonstrated between the two groups and are discussed in Chapter 3. As was observed by Sir William Gull some anorectics will, from time to time, gorge themselves. Garfinkel, Moldofsky and Garner (1980) have used the presence of bulimia to classify cases of anorexia nervosa. Again, this is discussed later.

Summary

It is hoped that this brief historical account will have set the scene for the rest of the book. In many respects little has changed. The clinical descriptions of Morton, Gull and Lasegue are still valid today, and the mainstays of treatment remain those suggested by Gull. The patients are separated from their families, put to bed, and encouraged to eat. If medication is given it is usually with the same intention as Morton's, namely to stimulate the appetite or to relieve anxiety.

References

BERKMAN, J. M. (1930) Anorexia nervosa, anorexia, inanation, and low basal metabolic rate. *Am. J. Med. Sci.*, **180**, 411–424

BEUMONT, P. J. V., GEORGE, G. C. W. and SMART, D. E. (1976) *Psychol. Med.*, **6**, 617–622

BHANJI, S. and NEWTON, V. B. (1985) Richard Morton's account of 'nervous consumption'. *Int. J. Eating Disorders*, **4**, 589–595

BLISS, E. L. AND BRANCH, C. H. H. (1960) *Anorexia Nervosa: its History, Psychology, and Biology.* New York: Paul B. Hoeber Inc.

BRUCH, H. (1962) Perceptual and conceptual disturbances in anorexia nervosa. *Psychosom. Med.*, **24**, 187–194

BRUCH, H. (1966) Anorexia nervosa and its differential diagnosis. *J. Nerv. Ment. Dis.*, **141**, 555–566

BRUCKNER, W. J., WEIS, C. H. and LAVIETES, P. H. (1938) Anorexia nervosa and pituitary cachexia. *Am. J. Med. Sci.*, **196**, 663–673

ESCAMILLA, R. F. and LISSER, H. (1942) Simmonds' disease: a clinical study with review of the literature; differentiation from anorexia nervosa by statistical analysis of 595 cases, 101 of which were proved pathologically. *J. Clin. Endocrinol.*, **2**, 65–96

GARFINKEL, P. E., MOLDOFSKY, H. and GARNER, D. M. (1980) The heterogeneity of anorexia nervosa: bulimia as a distinct subgroup. *Arch. Gen. Psychiatry*, **37**, 1036–1040

GOULD, M. G. and PYLE, W. L. (1901) *Anomalies and Curiosities of Medicine. Popular Edition.* London: W. B. Saunders & Co.

GULL, W. W. (1873) Anorexia hysterica (apepsia hysterica). *Br. Med. J.*, ii, 527–528

GULL, W. W. (1874) Anorexia nervosa (apepsia hysterica, anorexia hysterica). *Trans. Clin. Soc. Lond.*, **7**, 22–28

HAMMOND, W. A. (1879) *Fasting Girls: their Physiology and Psychology.* New York: G. P. Putnam's Sons

KAUFMAN, M. R. and HEIMAN, M. (1964) *Evolution of Psychosomatic Concepts*, pp. 143–155. New York: International Universities Press

KAY, D. W. K. and LEIGH, D. (1954) The natural history, treatment and prognosis of anorexia nervosa, based on a study of 38 patients. *J. Ment. Sci.*, **100**, 411–431

KING, A. (1963) Primary and secondary anorexia nervosa syndromes. *Br. J. Psychiatry*, **109**, 470–479

LASEGUE, C. (1873) De l'anorexie hysterique. *Arch. Gen. Med.*, **21**, 385–403

MCSHERRY, J. A. (1985) Was Mary, Queen of Scots, anorexic? *Scott. Med. J.*, **30**, 243–245

MEXIO, P. (1613) *The Treasurie of Auncient and Moderne Times*, pp. 547–552. London: Jaggard

MEYER, J.-E. (1961) Das Syndrom der Anorexia nervosa. *Arch. Psychiatr. Z. Neurol.*, **202**, 31–59

MORGAN, H. G. (1977) Fasting girls and our attitudes to them. *Br. Med. J.*, ii, 1652–55

MORTON, R. (1689) *Phthisologia: Sue Exercitationes de Phthisi*, pp. 4–11. London: S. Smith

MORTON, R. (1694) *Phthisologia: Or a Treatise of Consumptions*, pp. 4–10. London: S. Smith and B. Walford

NAISH, J. M. (1979) Problems of deception in medical practice. *Lancet*, ii, 139–142

NEMIAH, J. C. (1958) Anorexia nervosa: fact and theory. *Am. J. Dig. Dis.*, **3**, 249–274

RYLE, J. A. (1936) Anorexia nervosa. *Lancet*, ii, 893–895

SHEEHAN, H. L. and SUMMERS, V. K. (1949) The syndrome of hypopituitarism. *Q. J. Med.*, **18**, 319–378

SHELDON, J. H. (1939) Discussion on anorexia nervosa. *Proc. R. Soc. Med.*, **32**, 738–741

SILVERMAN, J. A. (1983) Richard Morton, 1637–1698 limner of anorexia nervosa: his life and times. *J. Am. Med. Assoc.*, **250**, 2830–2832

SIMMONDS, M. (1914) Ueber Hypophysisshwond mit Todlichen ausgane. *Dtsch. Med. Wochenschr.*, **1**, 322–323

YEARSLEY, M. (1935) *Le Roy est Mort: An Account of the Deaths of the Rulers of England*, pp. 44–45. London: John Heritage

Chapter 2

Aetiology

There are many opinions concerning the possible causes of anorexia nervosa. The physicians who provided the earlier description of the disorder were content to ascribe it to emotional troubles and leave it at that. Psychiatrists and those with an interest in neurophysiology and endocrinology have pursued the matter further. So far, no generally accepted view has emerged, but those theories deriving from psychiatry and psychology have attracted considerable support. The alternative opinion, that anorexia nervosa is primarily a somatic disorder, has its advocates, but they are very much in the minority.

Psychological theories

The earliest psychiatric approach to anorexia nervosa derived from psychoanalysis. Freud did not publish any case histories of anorexia nervosa, but he did mention that a neurotic fear of sexual activity occurred in some girls around the time of puberty and expressed itself as a loss of appetite (Freud, 1918, translated 1955). Broadly speaking, psychoanalytical theories regarding anorexia nervosa were of two types (Nemiah, 1958): one stressed unconscious or overt beliefs that impregnation could occur through the mouth; the other emphasized an intense, and sometimes mutual, dependency of the child on the mother, which was associated with the perpetuation of infantile attitudes and behaviour.

Later theories laid emphasis on the family as a whole and not just the patient and, furthermore, relegated anorexia to the status of a secondary and inconstant symptom. The paramount feature was seen as an intense desire to control the shape and size of the body. Three of the most popular theories are set out below. For a fuller account and discussion the reader is referred to Dally and Gomez (1979) and to Garfinkel and Garner (1982).

Hilde Bruch (1962) described three fundamental aspects of anorexia nervosa. The first of these is an inability to appreciate the need to be adequately nourished. The second is a disturbance of body image perception, which causes the patient to be unable to perceive how thin she really is. Finally, there is an intense feeling of ineffectiveness. The last, which is seen as central to the disorder, stems from the way the parents have treated their daughter. With the best will in the world they do everything for her. They select her friends, choose her school regardless of her abilities, and generally see to it that she gets what they regard as the best. In return, they expect unswerving gratitude, loyalty and affection. As a result the unfortunate girl comes to regard herself not as an individual, but as her parents' private property. In the end she protests by adopting an attitude of self-control and, in anorexia nervosa, carries it to the extreme. Bruch's views have important implications for treatment, since any method based on coercion, no matter how well-intentioned or benignly expressed, is unlikely in the long run to be of much benefit.

Whereas Bruch stressed a desire for autonomy, others hold to another popular theory in which they see anorexia nervosa as a means of avoiding independence and its consequences. A number of authors, in particular Minuchin, Rosman and Baker (1978) and Selvini Palazzoli (1974), writing from the standpoint of family therapy, have described families in which there are many overt and covert alliances. The intention, at least on the surface, is to create a healthy sense of mutual security, but only dependence develops. Faced with the biological signals of impending adulthood, and thence emancipation, the girl panics and tries to obliterate these. One method which is readily available to her is by drastically reducing her body weight.

The third theory holds that another family arrangement may lead to anorexia nervosa (Crisp, 1983). Here the relationship between the parents is unsatisfactory and unsatisfying, and a divorce or separation may happen once the children are old enough to look after themselves. The daughter senses what is going on and realizes that in order to keep the family together she must remain a dependent child for as long as she can. Faced with the adolescent growth spurt she then develops a weight phobia and starves herself.

It has been suggested that current social attitudes may explain not only the apparent increase in anorexia nervosa, but also its predilection for the adolescent middle-class female. Thinness in women has become equated with personal and professional success (Garner *et al.*, 1980). Many young women now have the option of a career instead of marriage or child-rearing. Hence examinations have become more important to them. Mills (1976) drew attention to the relationship between pre-examination study and the onset of anorexia nervosa, and a significant number of our patients became ill while studying for Advanced-level examinations (Mattingly and Bhanji, 1982). The attitude toward sexual activity is more permissive and means of contraception are more readily available, thus posing a threat to the sexually insecure young girl. Finally, the attitude of male-dominated society toward women is not dissimilar to that of parents to daughters as described by Bruch. Orbach (1985) has argued persuasively along these lines.

Somatic theories

The relationship between physical illness in general and anorexia nervosa has been explored by Patton, Wood and Johnson-Sabine (1986) who investigated over 300 cases and found that, in comparison with their control patients, the anorectics had a higher incidence of remote and recent severe physical disorders. The authors were not convinced of a direct causal association, but suggested that physical illness might increase the risk by generating an atmosphere of morbid concern within the family.

Particular interest has been devoted to hypothalamic or midbrain tumours and chromosome abnormalities. The first account of anorexia nervosa arising in Turner's syndrome was that provided by Pitts and Guze (1963). Although a number of other reports have since appeared, it remains debatable whether or not the concurrence of these conditions is greater or less than expected through chance (Garfinkel and Garner, 1982). Whatever the final view, the possibility that chromosome anomalies may predispose those afflicted towards anorexia nervosa has been further raised by recent reports of this condition in Down's syndrome (Cottrell and Crisp, 1984) and in a patient with Klinefelter's syndrome (Hindler and Norris, 1986).

Hypothalamic damage

Over 30 years ago it was shown that bilateral lesions of the lateral hypothalamus of laboratory rats could result in life-threatening avoidance of food (Anand and Brobeck, 1951). However, Stricker and Andersen (1980) have compared the lateral hypothalamic syndrome in animals with anorexia nervosa, but concluded that the only common factor was the loss of weight. On the other hand, there have been a number of reports of patients who have been diagnosed as having anorexia nervosa and later been found to have hypothalamic or midbrain tumours. The first convincing case was actually one of our earlier patients (Lewin, Mattingly and Millis, 1972). She was a 25-year-old nurse with a history of secondary amenorrhoea and weight loss due to avoidance of carbohydrate foods. There appeared to be strong psychological causes and there seemed no doubt that she had anorexia nervosa. Five days after her admission she developed spontaneous hypoglycaemia and went into coma, dying 3 weeks later from a salmonella septicaemia. At autopsy she was found to have a small hypothalamic astrocytoma. It was this experience that convinced us that some hypothalamic disturbance could be involved in the pathogenesis of this disease.

Further cases have since been described. An emaciated 22-year-old girl who presented in coma was reported the following year (Daly and Nabarro, 1973). There was a long history of obsession with her weight and dieting. At autopsy an atypical hypothalamic pinealoma was found. Rohmer, Ebtinger and Bronstein (1975) described a 15-year-old girl with a disturbed family background and an immature personality who had a 3-month history of vomiting, anorexia, apathy, loss of weight, and amenorrhoea. Neurological examination was normal on admission, but 5 months later evidence of raised intracranial pressure appeared. Unfortunately, it proved impossible to remove the medulloblastoma in the fourth ventricle which was responsible.

Heron and Johnston (1976) reported a male aged 24 years with persistent weight loss. His history revealed a number of emotional stresses and an overprotective mother. He was regarded as suffering from anorexia nervosa, and treated with behaviour therapy which was partially successful. Some months later he was admitted to hospital in a semi-comatose state and was found to have an ectopic hypothalamic pinealoma. White, Kelly and Dorman (1977) gave an account of a 15-year-old boy who had lost weight and had a long history of behaviour problems. Psychotherapy was started but the parents took him away. A few weeks later he became disorientated and dehydrated. Subsequent investigation revealed a large midline glioma in the region of the third ventricle. This was operated on and the appetite returned to normal, although the patient continued to be troubled by depression.

In 1982 Climo described a girl aged 22 years who was brought into hospital for long-term psychotherapy for schizophrenia. Her progress was stormy and after being particularly upset she vowed to stop eating. Some months afterwards she developed abdominal pain and a craving for sugar in spite of a fear of becoming fat. She also developed secondary amenorrhoea. During her third year of psychotherapy her discomfort eased and she gained weight. While preparations were being made for her discharge she developed a headache. Investigation revealed a craniopharyngioma. Weller and Weller (1982) reported an 11-year-old girl with typical features of anorexia nervosa, the clinical diagnosis having been made by no less than four child psychiatrists. She was found to have an infiltrating tumour of the hypothalamus and, after radiotherapy, her anorectic symptoms disappeared.

The case described by Goldney (1978) is particularly instructive. A 28-year-old married woman with a 5-year-old daughter was admitted to hospital with the diagnosis of hysteria and a history of previous treatment for anorexia nervosa and hysterical blindness. Following curettage for a missed abortion some 4 years beforehand, she began to lose weight and her periods ceased. She was seen by a gynaecologist who after some hesitation diagnosed anorexia nervosa. After psychiatric, further gynaecological, and finally medical assessment, during which her demanding nature was commented on, the diagnosis of anorexia nervosa was at last agreed upon. A year before her final admission to hospital the patient complained of increasing blindness. Ophthalmological examination showed no objective signs and it was thought that her sight was better than claimed. A neurological assessment was suggested but not undertaken. Some months later she was admitted to a psychiatric hospital where she proved uncooperative, demanding, generally antagonistic, and would request drinks at inappropriate times. Eventually optic atrophy was discovered and organic pathology finally accepted. This was all to no avail as shortly afterwards she died with an inoperable craniopharyngioma. The author comments that in retrospect the history was compatible with a craniopharyngioma, and it was largely the patient's manner that led to the erroneous diagnosis of anorexia nervosa. As autopsies are now rarely carried out on patients dying in psychiatric hospitals, it is tempting to speculate on how many others met with similar fates.

As is discussed in greater detail in Chapter 11, many if not all cases of anorexia nervosa show evidence of hypothalamic dysfunction. Temperature regulation is sometimes impaired, there may be failure to produce appropriately dilute or concentrated urine, and in about one-third of cases the amenorrhoea precedes any weight loss. There is much debate as to whether these changes point to a hypothalamic cause of anorexia nervosa or are merely consequences of starvation.

Neurophysiology

Other theories relevant to a somatic basis for anorexia nervosa stem from recent advances in neurophysiology. Mawson (1974) argued that feeding was associated with activation of subcortical dopaminergic or noradrenergic systems, and inhibition of cholinergic systems. In satiety the opposite applied. He regarded anorexia nervosa as due to progressive depletion of brain noradrenaline, dopamine, or both and suggested that their precursor, L-dopa, might be a useful form of treatment. By contrast, Barry and Klawans (1976) put forward a case for increased dopaminergic activity within the hypothalamus. The hypothalamus undergoes a number of important changes in function during puberty and adolescence, which are more marked in the female. They therefore regarded their hypothesis as consistent with the characteristic sex and age distribution and postulated a defect in negative feedback control. They suggested that either dopamine antagonists or L-dopa might reverse the symptoms.

The first study of catecholamine metabolism in anorectics was that of Halmi et al. (1978). They investigated 25 cases, but unfortunately some had already been given psychotropic drugs which may have affected their findings. The urinary excretion of the major metabolite of brain noradrenaline, 3-methoxy-4-hydroxy-phenylglycol (MHPG) was lower in the anorectics than in the controls, both before and after refeeding. Gross *et al.* (1979) found that plasma noradrenaline levels were also lower in anorectics than in normal control patients, but did not differ after recovery. Plasma tyrosine levels and the activity of dopamine beta-hydroxylase were normal throughout. By contrast, the urinary excretion of MHPG and homovanillic acid (HVA), an important brain dopamine metabolite, was reduced and tended to increase with treatment. Their patients were treated with behaviour therapy and thus a drug effect could not be held responsible. The low MHPG excretion in untreated anorectics was confirmed by Gerner and Gwirtsman (1981) and Abraham, Beumont and Cobbin (1981). Van Loon (1980) reported that in addition to serum noradrenaline concentrations, those of dopamine and adrenaline were also reduced. Riederer, Toifl and Kruzic (1982) measured the urinary excretion of the serotonin metabolite 5-hydroxyindole acetic acid (5-HIAA) as well as that of a variety of central and peripheral metabolites of noradrenaline and dopamine. Levels were decreased in comparison to those in their control group, and increased in the four cases who were re-investigated after treatment. The increased excretion in the recovered patients correlated with the increase in weight.

Kaye *et al.* (1984a) investigated the cerebrospinal fluid (CSF) concentrations of HVA, noradrenaline and 5-HIAA, and the blood levels of tryptophan, tyrosine and phenylalanine in 10 anorectics. Their findings suggested that the metabolism of serotonin and dopamine is decreased when weight is low. By contrast, CSF levels of noradrenaline were normal throughout treatment. In a further study, bulimic and non-bulimic anorectics were compared (Kaye *et al.*, 1984b). After recovery the non-bulimic cases had higher CSF concentrations of 5-HIAA than those of the bingers, but there were no differences with regard to HVA.

Monoamine oxidase plays a crucial role in the catabolism of a wide variety of monoamines. The discovery that blood platelets contain this enzyme has facilitated research into its activity. Biederman *et al.* (1984) investigated platelet monoamine activity in anorexia nervosa, and found it to be reduced, but only in those cases who, in addition to having anorexia, were suffering from a concomitant depressive illness.

We know of no published studies of brain histochemistry in those who died as the result of anorexia nervosa or were subjected to psychosurgery. However, we were able to re-examine the hypothalamic tumour from our patient. Sections from the original tissue block were deparaffinized, subjected to formalin vapour for 30 minutes, and examined under ultraviolet light for catecholamines. The tumour was found to contain substantially more catecholamine-secreting neurons than the surrounding tissue.

Those familiar with the research into the role monoamine neurotransmitters play in the manic depressive disorders will be well aware of the technical and methodological problems involved. We suspect the same difficulties will apply to anorexia nervosa. A major problem is the recent discovery that there are far more substances involved in neurotransmission than just acetylcholine and the monoamines. For example, Kaye *et al.* (1982) measured total opioid activity in five underweight anorectics; eight anorectics who had recovered their weight, of whom four had resumed menstruation; and seven healthy women of comparable age. None of the subjects were taking medication. The mean level of CSF opioid activity, measured as beta-endorphin equivalents, was significantly higher in the untreated anorectics. Some of the subjects completed a rating scale assessing distress associated with various aspects of eating. The scores fell with treatment, but did not correlate with changes in opioid activity.

During the last 20 years it has been discovered that a number of hormones are present both in the gut and within the brain, particularly the hypothalamus.

Thyrotropin releasing hormone (TRH) and anorexigenic peptide appear to inhibit feeding as well as affect gastrointestinal secretions. Glucagon, bombesin, somatostatin, gastrin, and cholecystokinin have all been proposed as satiety factors, and the last two may be involved in the control of vomiting. Vasoactive intestinal polypeptide may effect sexual arousal, somatostatin may lead to increased motor activity, and neurotensin can cause hypotension and cold extremities. It may well be that such substances act as the common factor between the eating disorders and the emotional, behavioural and physical changes which accompany them.

Alderdice et al. (1985) have measured fasting and postprandial blood levels of glucose and a number of hormones in eight cases of anorexia nervosa and a group of age and sex-matched healthy controls. In the fasting state the mean levels of glucose, insulin and pancreatic glucagon were lower in the anorectics. After a standard meal (50 g carbohydrate, 20 g fat and 18 g protein) the patients showed impaired glucose tolerance, and a reduced and delayed insulin response. The release of gastric inhibitory polypeptide (GIP), normally a sensitive responder to carbohydrates, was reduced, but the secretion of pancreatic polypeptide was augmented. The anorectics had higher gastrin levels, but not to a significant extent. It was suggested that both the low glucose and insulin levels may have resulted from reduced secretion of pancreatic glucagon. The diminished GIP response to the meal could explain the muted insulin response and rise in blood glucose. The latter could be detected by the hypothalamus and the patient would then feel satiated. This model does not rule out hypothalamic pathology, but the authors suggested that the primary abnormality in anorexia nervosa could be the gut response to carbohydrates. By contrast, Dixon et al. (1985) found the release of GIP to be increased in anorectics after a meal.

Trygstad et al. (1978) examined the urinary peptide chromatographic patterns in 25 cases of anorexia nervosa and found them to be of four different types. One appeared to characterize those anorectics with evidence of hypothalamic dysfunction. This group in particular had an earlier onset of symptoms, delayed growth and development, and primary amenorrhoea. They isolated an anorexigenic peptide (pryoGlu-His-GlyOH) which induced anorexia and weight loss when injected into mice (Reichelt et al., 1978). It was suggested that this peptide was secreted by the hypothalamus. Konturek et al. (1981) compared the effects of anorexigenic peptide and the structurally similar peptide TRH on the gastrointestinal secretions of conscious dogs. Both substances inhibited feeding and gastrointestinal secretory activity, particularly that of the pancreas.

Summary

Although the psychological theories concerning the causes of anorexia nervosa are by far the most popular, we have concentrated deliberately on the physiological abnormalities which have been found in some of these patients. This is by no means intended to disparage the former, but to draw attention to the latter. Most doctors would agree that psychological stresses usually trigger off anorexia nervosa, but there are some patients in whom the only precipitant appears to be over-energetic dieting. However, what is debatable is whether the physical changes that result are secondary to starvation or to a subtle disturbance in the neuroendocrine system in vulnerable young people. The point of view that is taken will inevitably affect the management.

References

ABRAHAM, S. F., BEUMONT, P. J. V. and COBBIN, D. M. (1981) Catecholamine metabolism and body weight in anorexia nervosa. *Br. J. Psychiatry*, **138**, 244–247

ALDERDICE, J. T., DINSMORE, W. W., BUCHANAN, K. D. and ADAMS, C. (1985) Gastrointestinal hormones in anorexia nervosa. *J. Psychiatr. Res.*, **19**, 207–213

ANAND, B. K. and BROBECK, J. R. (1951) Localization of a 'feeding centre' in the hypothalamus of the rat. *Proc. Soc. Exp. Biol. Med.*, **77**, 323–324

BARRY, V. C. and KLAWANS, H. L. (1976) On the role of dopamine in the pathophysiology of anorexia nervosa. *J. Neural. Trans.*, **38**, 107–122

BIEDERMAN, J., RIVINUS, T. M., HERZOG, D. B., FERBER, R. A., HARPER, G. P., ORSULAK, P. J. *et al.* (1984) Platelet MAO activity in anorexia nervosa patients with and without a major depressive disorder. *Am. J. Psychiatry*, **141**, 1244–1247

BRUCH, H. (1962) Perceptual and conceptual disturbances in anorexia nervosa. *Psychosom. Med.*, **24**, 187–194

CLIMO, L. H. (1982) Anorexia nervosa associated with hypothalamic tumor: the search for clinical-pathological correlations. *Psychiatr. J. Univ. Ottawa*, **7**, 20–25

COTTRELL, D. J. and CRISP, A. H. (1984) Anorexia nervosa in Down's syndrome—a case report. *Br. J. Psychiatry*, **138**, 244–247

CRISP, A. H. (1983) Anorexia nervosa. *Br. Med. J.*, **287**, 855–858

DALLY, P. and GOMEZ, J. (1979) *Anorexia Nervosa*. London: William Heinemann Medical Books Ltd

DALY, J. J. and NABARRO, J. N. D. (1973) A case of anorexia. *Br. Med. J.*, i, 156–161

DIXON, K. N., O'DORISIO, T. M., ZIPF, W. and CATALAND, S. (1985) Gastric inhibitory polypeptide (GIP) in anorexia nervosa. *Int. J. Eating Disorders*, **4**, 597–604

FREUD, S. (1918) Aus der Geschichte einer Infantilen Neurose. In *The Standard Edition of the Complete Psychological Works of Sigmund Freud, Vol. XVII*, translated by J. Stracey, 1955. London: The Hogarth Press

GARFINKEL, P. E. and GARNER, D. M. (1982) *Anorexia Nervosa: A Multidimensional Perspective*. New York: Brunner/Mazel

GARNER, D. M., GARFINKEL, P. E., SCHWARTZ, D. and THOMPSON, M. (1980) Cultural expectations of thinness in women. *Psychol. Rep.*, **47**, 483–491

GERNER, R. H. and GWIRTSMAN, H. E. (1981) Abnormalities of dexamethasone suppression test and urinary MHPG in anorexia nervosa. *Am. J. Psychiatry*, **138**, 650–653

GOLDNEY, R. D. (1978) Craniopharyngioma simulating anorexia nervosa. *J. Nerv. Ment. Dis.*, **166**, 135–138

GROSS, H. A., LAKE, R. C., EBERT, M. H., ZIEGLER, M. G. and KOPIN, I. J. (1979) Catecholamine metabolism and primary anorexia nervosa. *J. Clin. Endocrinol. Metab.*, **49**, 805–809

HALMI, K. A., DEKIRMENTJIAN, H., DAVIS, J. M., CASPER, R. and GOLDBERG, S. (1978) Catecholamine metabolism in anorexia nervosa. *Arch. Gen. Psychiatry*, **35**, 458–460

HERON, G. B. and JOHNSTON, D. A. (1976) Hypothalamic tumor presenting as anorexia nervosa. *Am. J. Psychiatry*, **133**, 580–582

HINDLER, C. G. and NORRIS, D. L. (1986) A case of anorexia nervosa with Klinefelter's syndrome. *Br. J. Psychiatry*, **149**, 659–660

KAYE, W. H., EBERT, M. H., GWIRTSMAN, H. E. and WEISS, S. R. (1984b) Differences in brain serotonergic metabolism between nonbulimic and bulimic patients with anorexia nervosa. *Am. J. Psychiatry*, **141**, 1598–1601

KAYE, W. H., EBERT, M. H., RALEIGH, M. and LAKE, C. R. (1984a) Abnormalities in CNS monoamine metabolism in anorexia nervosa. *Arch. Gen. Psychiatry*, **41**, 350–355

KAYE, W. H., PICKAR, D., NABER, D. and EBERT, M. H. (1982) Cerebrospinal fluid opioid activity in anorexia nervosa. *Am. J. Psychiatry*, **193**, 643–645

KONTUREK, S. J., TASLER, J., JAWOREK, J., DOBRZANSKA, M., COY, D. H. and SCHALLY, A. V. (1981) Comparison of TRH and anorexigenic peptide on food intake and gastrointestinal secretions. *Peptides*, **2** (suppl. 2), 235–240

LEWIN, K., MATTINGLY, D. and MILLIS, R. R. (1972) Anorexia nervosa associated with hypothalamic tumour. *Br. Med. J.*, ii, 629–630

MATTINGLY, D. and BHANJI, S. (1982) The diagnosis of anorexia nervosa. *J. R. Coll. Physicians Lond.*, **16**, 191–194

MAWSON, A. R. (1974) Anorexia nervosa and the regulation of intake: a review. *Psychol. Med.*, **4**, 289–308

MILLS, I. H. (1978) The disease of failure of coping. *Practitioner*, **217**, 529–538

MINUCHIN, S., ROSMAN, B. L. and BAKER, L. (1978) *Psychosomatic Families: Anorexia Nervosa in Context.* Cambridge, Mass.: Harvard University Press

NEMIAH, J. C. (1958) Anorexia nervosa: fact and theory. *Am. J. Dig. Dis.*, **3**, 249–274

ORBACH, A. (1985) Visibility/invisibility: social considerations in anorexia nervosa—a feminist perspective. In *Theory and Treatment of Anorexia Nervosa and Bulimia*, edited by S. W. Emmett, pp. 127–138. New York: Brunner/Mazel

PATTON, G. C., WOOD, K. and JOHNSON-SABINE, E. (1986) Physical illness: a risk factor in anorexia nervosa. *Br. J. Psychiatry*, **149**, 756–759

PITTS, F. N. and GUZE, S. B. (1963) Anorexia nervosa and gonadal dysgenesis (Turner's syndrome). *Am. J. Psychiatry*, **119**, 1100–1102

REICHELT, K. L., FOSS, S., TRYGSTAD, J. H. and EDMINSON, P. D. (1978) Humoral control of appetite—II. Purification and characterization of an anorexigenic peptide from human urine. *Neuroscience*, **3**, 1207–1211

RIEDERER, F., TOIFL, K. and KRUZIC, P. (1982) Excretion of biogenic amine metabolites in anorexia nervosa. *Clin. Chim. Acta*, **123**, 27–32

ROHMER, A., EBTINGER, R. and BRONSTEIN, J. (1975) Fauste anorexie mentale vraie tumeur du IV ventricle. *Rev. Neuropsychiatr. Infantile*, **23**, 191–193

SELVINI PALAZZOLI, M. (1974) *Self-starvation: from the Intrapsychic to the Transpersonal Approach to Anorexia Nervosa.* London: Chaucer Publishing Co. Ltd

STRICKER, E. M. and ANDERSEN, A. E. (1980) The lateral hypothalamic syndrome: a comparison with the symptoms of anorexia nervosa. *Life Sci.*, **26**, 1927–1934

TRYGSTAD, O., FOSS, S., EDMINSON, P. D., JOHANSEN, J. H. and REICHELT, K. L. (1978) Humoral control of appetite: a urinary anorexigenic peptide. Chromatographic patterns of urinary peptides in anorexia nervosa. *Acta Endocrinol.*, **89**, 196–208

VAN LOON, G. R. (1980) Abnormal catecholamine mechanisms in hypothalamic-pituitary disorders. *Metabolism*, **29** (suppl. 1), 1198–1202

WELLER, R. A. and WELLER, E. B. (1982) Anorexia nervosa in a patient with an infiltrating tumor of the hypothalamus. *Am. J. Psychiatry*, **139**, 824–825

WHITE, J. H., KELLY, P. and DORMAN, K. (1977) Clinical picture of atypical anorexia nervosa associated with hypothalamic tumour. *Am. J. Psychiatry*, **134**, 323–325

Chapter 3

Clinical features

Descriptions of anorexia nervosa usually begin by stating that the overwhelming majority of cases are intelligent, overconscientious, white females who come from middle-class families. However, most of these studies have been carried out in Europe, North America or South Africa. Whereas this stereotype still applies to most patients, it appears from a number of sources that, although the majority of anorectics are still female, the age range and social class distribution are becoming wider (Garfinkel and Garner, 1982). Anorexia nervosa has also been occasionally described in the mentally handicapped. For example, Gift, Strauss and Ritzler (1978) measured the intelligence of 188 psychiatric inpatients and found one case of anorexia nervosa among the 22 patients with an intelligence quotient of 85 or less. The first detailed account, however, was that provided by Hurley and Sovner (1979) who described a 15-year-old mentally handicapped girl suffering from anorexia nervosa, and went on to suggest that the prevalence of this disorder among those of limited intellect may be higher than generally thought. More recently, Cottrell and Crisp (1984) have reported anorexia nervosa in a case of Down's syndrome.

Anorectics are now being reported to come from a variety of racial and national backgrounds: for example anorexia nervosa appears to be as common in Japan as in the western world (Suematsu *et al.*, 1985). Patients have been recorded in Nigeria (Nwaefuna, 1981), Zimbabwe (Buchan and Gregory, 1984) and among West Indians living in London (Thomas and Szmukler, 1985). Time will tell whether these epidemiological changes derive from altering sociocultural attitudes, or to more widespread knowledge of this condition.

Definitions

The diagnosis of those conditions in which psychological abnormality is a prominent feature is very much a matter of subjective interpretation of what the patient chooses to say and how he or she behaves. In recent years there have been a number of attempts to standardize psychiatric diagnoses by providing objective criteria. Among the most widely used are those of Feighner *et al.* (1972), the World Health Organization (1978) and the American Psychiatric Association (1980).

So far as anorexia nervosa is concerned, these all emphasize perverse eating behaviour which stems from an irrational desire to be thin. The resulting loss of weight may be accompanied by other physical changes; of these prominence is given to secondary amenorrhoea. It is usually, but not always, stipulated that the patient must be free of other illness which could result in loss of appetite or weight. Although they have done much towards improving the validity of research findings, some of the recommended criteria have been criticized by clinicians as being too rigid. For example, many would disagree with the suggestion of Feighner *et al.* that the diagnosis of anorexia nervosa should only be made if the illness begins before the age of 25 years and has resulted in the patient losing one-quarter of her weight. In a number of series a weight loss of more than 10% of the premorbid weight has been taken as an adequate criterion.

Weight loss

The most striking clinical feature, and that which most commonly leads to referral for treatment or investigation, is loss of weight. This is usually reported as beginning after dieting to counter the effects of perhaps too hearty an appetite or the natural development of adolescent 'puppy fat'. Teasing by her peers is common and may coincide with a variety of other emotional stresses which appear to act as precipitating factors.

A substantial number of our earlier cases were worried about impending school examinations or were unhappy at school. Just under 10% had been upset by the recent death of a close relative, and slightly more came from families where the parents were divorced or living apart (Mattingly and Bhanji, 1982).

The dieting, which mainly involves the avoidance of carbohydrate foods, often begins as a group activity. However, whereas the healthy girls are able to stop once their weight reaches an appropriate level the anorectic is not. The reasons for this are little understood, but three psychological factors are thought by many to play a significant, if not vital, role.

The first is a disturbance of body image such that the girl remains convinced that she is still too fat. The diagnostic significance of body size overestimation is controversial: some regard it as being a necessary criterion, others as no more than a common but not specific finding (Halmi, 1983). Whatever the importance of body image disturbance, accounts of anorexia nervosa in the blind and severely poor sighted suggest that being unable to see one's body does not prevent the illness from occurring (Bruch, 1983; Vandereycken, 1986; Yager, Watton and Ma, 1986). The second factor is a morbid fear that resuming anything like a healthy food intake will result in obesity. Thirdly, the patient is unable to accept any suggestion that her dieting has gone too far and that she is suffering from its harmful effects.

Distinguishing between the potential anorectic and the healthy dieter is not an easy matter. It has been noted, however, that the healthy girl will widen her social activities as she becomes thinner. On the other hand, the girl who will go on to develop the illness becomes less sociable and is interested only in food, her weight and her schoolwork. So far as the last is concerned she may show no personal pride in her achievements, but will be pleased that she has done her duty and satisfied her parents.

Finally, in addition to dieting there may be other changes in eating habits. For example, the girl may insist on preparing her own meals and may become increasingly reluctant to eat in company. If she cannot avoid eating with others, food is surreptitiously disposed of or smeared around the plate so that it appears as though she has eaten most of it.

Exercise is a common and fashionable means of achieving weight loss, and many clinicians have been impressed by the vitality of even their most emaciated patients. It is widely assumed that the hyperactivity of the anorectic is a deliberate attempt to burn up calories. However, there are other explanations. The most popular is that overactivity helps the patient to convince others that she is not ill. A contrary view is that of Kron *et al.* (1978) who suggested that hyperactivity is a primary and enduring feature of anorexia nervosa. They based their conclusion on a study of 33 patients, in 15 of whom follow-up data were available. In 21 of their 25 cases who were hyperactive on admission this had commenced before any dieting or weight loss. Of the anorectics who were observed after treatment, eight remained overactive even though their weight had been restored. The authors reported that before and after the period of weight loss excessive physical activity was purposeful, organized, well-planned and expressed in a socially acceptable fashion such as jogging or ballet lessons. By contrast, when their weight was low the patients described their overactivity as compulsive, incessant, disorganized and aimless.

A more ominous habit is the use of self-induced vomiting or the abuse of emetics, purgatives or diuretics in order to avoid weight gain. Because of the secrecy about their eating habits it is difficult to judge the extent to which anorectics indulge in such behaviour. In our experience a number of those who clearly vomit will deny the practice or claim that it occurs spontaneously. Those who abuse laxatives will rarely admit it or will state that they only take them occasionally for constipation. Beumont, George and Smart (1976) carried out a detailed study of 31 female patients and came to the conclusion that nearly half were vomiters and purgers. The latter group were more likely to have been obese before their illness and so the degree of weight loss was often less obvious. The prognosis of these patients was poorer, and they were more prone to medical complications.

A final, and rarely used, means of controlling weight is to take advantage of any concurrent disease which may itself result in weight loss. This has been reported in a number of anorectics who also suffer from insulin-dependent diabetes (Roland and Bhanji, 1982) and in a chronic anorectic who refused to allow anyone to treat her thyrotoxicosis (Rolla, El-Hajj and Goldstein 1986).

The extent of weight loss in the anorectic patient depends on a variety of factors. These include the degree of success in concealing perverse eating habits and their effect; the latter is often dealt with by wearing loose-fitting clothes or the adoption of a hair style which makes the patient appear taller. The careful application of facial make-up may mask sunken cheeks, or even make them appear attractive. Much depends on the ability of the family to recognize what is going on and to persuade the patient to seek early medical advice.

Anorexia

Diminished appetite is one of the hallmarks of anorexia nervosa, although there is controversy as to whether this constitutes true anorexia or merely a perverse attitude towards certain fattening foods. Most patients claim they eat enough, but closer scrutiny reveals that they are deliberately avoiding carbohydrates. Paradoxically, many express an extreme interest in food, and some cases will on occasions have uncontrollable bouts of overeating (bulimia). Garfinkel, Moldofsky and Garner (1980) studied 141 patients of whom 48% had experienced episodes of bulimia. In a few the binging antedated or coincided with the loss of weight, but in the majority it did not commence until some months later. The bulimic patients were more likely to induce vomiting or abuse laxatives. They were more active sexually, and displayed a variety of impulsive acts. The latter included drug and alcohol abuse, theft, parasuicide and self-mutilation.

In view of their abnormal eating habits it is hardly surprising that many patients are troubled by epigastric discomfort and fullness after meals, and are constipated. These and other less prevalent consequences are discussed elsewhere in this book.

Amenorrhoea

Secondary amenorrhoea is usual, but the younger patients may never have menstruated. There is considerable disagreement as to whether the cessation of menstruation is due primarily to disturbed hypothalamic function or is secondary to weight loss. In support of the former view is the fact that amenorrhoea antedates any significant loss of weight in about one-third of cases. It has been suggested that anorectics whose amenorrhoea precedes or coincides with the onset of weight loss constitute a subgroup in whom a primary hypothalamic disturbance plays a greater aetiological role than emotional strain. If this were so it would be expected that those with early onset amenorrhoea would show less evidence of exposure to stress. Nineteen of our patients completed the Crown–Crisp Experiential Index, a measure of neurotic responses to stress (Crown and Crisp, 1966). The mean score in the eight with early onset amenorrhoea was 32.4, that of the 11 with amenorrhoea following weight loss was 50.9 ($P<0.05$). Unfortunately, the latter group contained a higher proportion of vomiters and purgers—a population of anorectics who are known to be more neurotic.

Many of those who regard amenorrhoea as a consequence of weight loss believe that it is triggered off when the body weight falls below a certain critical level. It is therefore assumed that the periods will rapidly return with the achievement of a normal body weight (Crisp and Stonehill, 1971; Frisch, 1977). That this is not always so was shown by Falk and Halmi (1982) who followed-up 40 treated anorectics and were unable to demonstrate a correlation between their weights one year later and whether or not menstruation had resumed. Most of those who were still amenorrhoeic in spite of having a normal weight had continued to be selective in their diets.

Physical signs

Examination reveals a thin and often emaciated body with marked depletion of body fat. Secondary sexual characteristics are usually well-preserved in postpubertal cases. Most authors say that the breasts are of normal size. Beck and Brochner-Mortensen (1954) were among the first to question this assumption, having found small breasts in 10 out of 13 patients. More recently, Warren and Vande Weile (1973) commented that the breasts may show some atrophy, and we have certainly seen significant breast atrophy in 13 women, most of whom had been ill for more than 4 years. Axillary and pubic hair are usually normal in amount and distribution. Scanty sexual hair was noted in only 5% of our cases.

The skin is often dry and pale in appearance. Acrocyanosis is common, and sometimes a yellow-orange discoloration of the palms and soles may be observed in those with hypercarotenaemia. Rarely the various skin manifestations of vitamin deficiency occur. Lanugo is frequently found, particularly on the trunk and limbs. According to Wright, Manwell and Merrett (1969) this is a distinguishing feature of anorexia nervosa, but most regard it as a non-specific affect of starvation. Dermatitis artefacta is sometimes seen in severely disturbed patients and was present in three of our cases.

Other signs which may be commonly encountered are bradycardia and hypotension. These, along with other physical manifestations and complications of anorexia nervosa are discussed in other chapters.

Anorexia nervosa in males

It would appear that a substantial proportion of doctors do not believe that anorexia nervosa occurs in males (Bhanji, 1979). In part this stems from insistence on amenorrhoea before the diagnosis can be made, and in part to a conviction that the underlying psychopathology is specific to the female. Beumont, Beardwood and Russell (1972) reviewed the literature and traced a total of 250 alleged male cases of anorexia nervosa. In the majority no firm evidence was presented to support the diagnosis. The authors were left with only 25 instances of probable anorexia nervosa, to which they added six of their own. In the same year, a further 13 cases were described by Crisp and Toms (1972). The majority view nowadays is that this disorder does occur in adolescent males but is uncommon. The main clinical features are unexplained weight loss and profound constipation.

Anorexia nervosa in older women

Anorexia nervosa rarely develops after the age of 25 years, but older patients have been described and we have seen a few. Ryle (1936) reported 13 women who became ill between the ages of 31 and 59 years. He regarded the precipitating factors as multiple and varied, but commonly included an operation, illness or the menopause. The physical and psychological findings were similar to those seen in the younger subjects. There are many other causes of anorexia and loss of weight in the middle-aged and elderly and the diagnosis of anorexia nervosa should only be entertained after thorough investigation has excluded organic disease and psychotic illness. For example, in common with others we believe that the 94- year-old patient described by Bernstein (1972) was in fact suffering from a depressive illness which responded to electroconvulsive therapy.

Summary

In this chapter we have described the major clinical features of anorexia nervosa and the controversy surrounding some of these. We believe that the diagnosis can and should be made in the majority of cases on the basis of the characteristic history and clinical findings. Unlike Sir William Gull we do not feel that excluding all other causes of weight loss is a necessary first step towards the recognition of the typical case. In the next chapter we provide a more detailed account of the patients in our own series.

References

AMERICAN PSYCHIATRIC ASSOCIATION (1980) *Diagnostic and Statistical Manual of Mental Disorders (Third Edition)*. Washington DC: APA

BECK, J. C. and BROCHNER-MORTENSEN, K. (1954) Observations on the prognosis in anorexia nervosa. *Acta Med. Scand.*, **149**, 409–430

BERNSTEIN, I. C. (1972) Anorexia nervosa: 94-year-old woman treated with electroshock. *Minn. Med.*, **55**, 552–553

BEUMONT, P. J. V., BEARDWOOD, C. J. and RUSSELL, G. F. M. (1972) The occurrence of the syndrome of anorexia nervosa in male subjects. *Psychol. Med.*, **2**, 216–231

BEUMONT, P. J. V., GEORGE, G. C. W. and SMART, D. E. (1976) 'Dieters' and 'vomiters and purgers' in anorexia nervosa. *Psychol. Med.*, **6**, 617–622

BHANJI, S. (1979) Anorexia nervosa: physicians' and psychiatrists' opinions and practice. *J. Psychosom. Res.*, **23**, 7–11

BRUCH, H. (1983) *Eating Disorders. Obesity, Anorexia Nervosa, and the Person Within*. New York: Basic Books

BUCHAN, T. and GREGORY, L. D. (1984) Anorexia nervosa in a black Zwimbabwean. *Br. J. Psychiatry*, **145**, 326–330

COTTRELL, D. J. and CRISP, A. H. (1984) Anorexia nervosa in Down's syndrome—a case report. *Br. J. Psychiatry*, **145**, 195–196

CRISP, A. H. and STONEHILL, E. (1971) Relationship between aspects of nutritional disturbance and menstrual activity in primary anorexia nervosa. *Br. Med. J.*, **3**, 149–151

CRISP, A. H. and TOMS, D. A. (1972) Primary anorexia nervosa or weight phobia in the male: report on 13 cases. *Br. Med. J.*, i, 334–338

CROWN, S. and CRISP, A. H. (1966) A short clinical diagnostic self-rating scale for psychoneurotic patients: the Middlesex Hospital questionnaire (MHQ). *Br. J. Psychiatry*, **112**, 917–923

FALK, J. R. and HALMI, K. A. (1982) Amenorrhea in anorexia nervosa: examination of the critical body weight hypothesis. *Biol. Psychiatry*, **17**, 799–806

FEIGHNER, J. P., ROBINS, E., GUZE, S., WOODRUFF, G. and MUNOZ, R. (1972) Diagnostic criteria for use in psychiatric research. *Arch. Gen. Psychiatry*, **26**, 57–63

FRISCH, R. E. (1977) Food intake, fatness, and reproductive ability. In *Anorexia Nervosa*, edited by R. A. Vigersky, pp. 149–161. New York: Raven Press

GARFINKEL, P. E. and GARNER, D. M. (1982) *Anorexia Nervosa: a Multidimensional Perspective*. New York: Brunner/Mazel

GARFINKEL, P. E., MOLDOFSKY, H. and GARNER, D. M. (1980) The heterogeneity of anorexia nervosa: bulimia as a distinct subgroup. *Arch. Gen. Psychiatry*, **37**, 1036–1040

GIFT, T. E., STRAUSS, J. S. and RITZLER, B. A. (1978) The failure to detect low IQ in psychiatric assessment. *Am. J. Psychiatry*, **135**, 345–349

HALMI, K. A. (1983) Anorexia nervosa and bulimia. *Psychosomatics*, **24**, 111–129

HURLEY, A. D. and SOVNER, R. (1979) Anorexia nervosa and mental retardation: a case report. *J. Clin. Psychiatry*, **40**, 480–482

KRON, L., KATZ, J. L., GORZYNSKI, G. and WEINER, H. (1978) Hyperactivity in anorexia nervosa: a fundamental clinical feature. *Compr. Psychiatry*, **19**, 438–440

MATTINGLY, D. and BHANJI, S. (1982) The diagnosis of anorexia nervosa. *J. R. Coll. Physicians Lond.*, **16**, 191–194

NWAEFUNA, A. (1981) Anorexia nervosa in a developing country. *Br. J. Psychiatry*, **138**, 270

ROLAND, J. M. and BHANJI, S. (1982) Anorexia nervosa occurring in patients with diabetes mellitus. *Postgrad. Med. J.*, **58**, 354–356

ROLLA, A. R., EL-HAJJ, G. A. and GOLDSTEIN, H. H. (1986) Untreated thyrotoxicosis as a manifestation of anorexia nervosa. *Am. J. Med.*, **81**, 163–165

RYLE, J. A. (1936) Anorexia nervosa. *Lancet*, ii, 893–899

SUEMATSU, H., ISHIKAWA, H., KUBOKI, T. and ITO, T. (1985) Statistical studies on anorexia nervosa in Japan: detailed clinical data on 1011 patients. *Psychother. Psychosom.*, **43**, 96–103

THOMAS, J. P. and SZMUKLER, G. I. (1985) Anorexia nervosa in patients of Afro-Caribbean extraction. *Br. J. Psychiatry*, **146**, 653–656

VANDEREYCKEN, W. (1986) Anorexia nervosa and visual impairment. *Compr. Psychiatry*, **27**, 545–548

WARREN, M. P. and VANDE WIELE, R. L. (1973) Clinical and metabolic features of anorexia nervosa. *Am. J. Obstet. Gynecol.*, **117**, 435–448

WORLD HEALTH ORGANIZATION (1978) *Mental Disorders: Glossary and Guide to their Classification in accordance with the Ninth Revision of the International Classification of Diseases.* Geneva: WHO

WRIGHT, W. S., MANWELL, M. K. C. and MERRETT, J. D. (1969) Anorexia nervosa: a discriminant function analysis. *Br. J. Psychiatry*, **115**, 829–831

YAGER, J., WATTON, C. A. and MA, L. (1986) Anorexia nervosa in a woman totally blind since the age of two. *Br. J. Psychiatry*, **149**, 506–509

Chapter 4

The authors' series

In 1982 we published the clinical and laboratory findings in a consecutive series of 91 cases of anorexia nervosa referred to one of us at a District General Hospital between 1966 and 1981 (Mattingly and Bhanji, 1982). Since then we have seen a further 64 cases, making a total of 155.

Diagnostic criteria

In the earliest cases the diagnosis was based on the traditional criteria of anorexia, weight loss, amenorrhoea and the absence of any physical illness to account for these signs. With the benefit of further experience it proved both possible and necessary to be more specific. All our patients showed the following features.

(1) Weight loss of at least 10% of the calculated optimum for sex, age and height as determined from standard tables or growth charts (Tanner and Whitehouse, 1975).
(2) Avoidance of carbohydrate foods. The term avoidance includes consumption and then riddance by vomiting or purgation as well as exclusion from the diet.
(3) Amenorrhoea of at least 3 months' duration, provided that the patient was not taking an oral contraceptive.
(4) The absence of any other psychiatric illness.
(5) The absence of any organic disease which could account for the weight loss.
(6) The characteristic physical appearance described below.

The patients

One hundred and fifty-one females and four males who fulfilled the above criteria were seen between May 1966 and April 1986. In approximately one-fifth the diagnosis of anorexia nervosa had not been considered by the referring doctor, usually the general practitioner. Three were suspected of having hyperthyroidism, one was thought to have Addison's disease, and one an insulinoma. Other diagnoses included malignancy and malabsorption.

The patients' ages when first seen ranged from 13 to 67 years, the overwhelming majority being less than 25 years old. *Figure 4.1* illustrates the ages at the onset of the loss of weight. The number of older patients was unexpected, particularly the one over 60 (Ramell and Brown, 1988). The great majority were single, 14 were married,

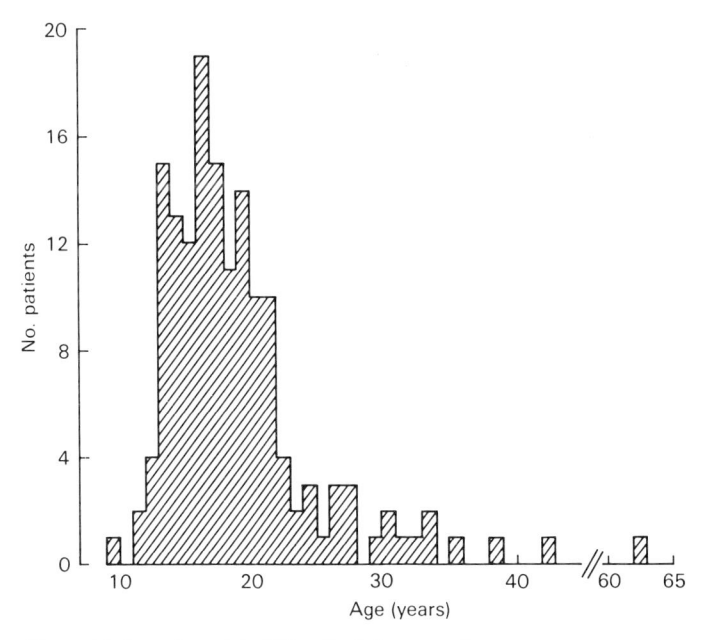

Figure 4.1 Age of onset in 155 patients in our series

four were divorced or separated, and there was one widow. The social class was recorded in 95, two-thirds of whom came from classes I or II.

In most of the patients their previous medical histories were uneventful. However, 24 were known or discovered to have a concurrent medical or surgical disorder. Five patients suffered from epilepsy, five had hirsutism and polycystic ovaries, two were insulin-dependent diabetics, and two had confirmed duodenal ulcers. Three patients had skin lesions due to dermatitis artefacta. One girl was mentally handicapped and another had Turner's syndrome. Other associated conditions included infarction of the right parietal lobe following a head injury, an arteriovenous malformation within the left temporal lobe, unilateral optic atrophy due to encephalitis in childhood, neurofibromatosis without cerebral involvement, a benign parotid tumour, fibrous dysplasia of a rib, congenital deformity of the right hand, and a colostomy following surgery for endometriosis. Finally, the singular case with a hypothalamic astrocytoma is described in some detail in Chapter 3.

Symptoms

All but one of the 155 patients acknowledged that they had lost weight. In the case who did not, her parents and general practitioner confirmed that she was becoming thinner. The duration of weight loss ranged from as little as 3 months to 20 years, but the majority had been losing weight for less than 2 years. Thirty-eight patients had been ill for longer than this, and included eight who had been anorectic for more than 10 years. Their weights on presentation ranged from 24.6 to 55.0 kg; this represented a loss of between 10 and 50% of their calculated optimum weight.

All the patients eventually admitted to avoiding carbohydrate food, but one-third

Table 4.1 Symptoms in 155 cases of anorexia nervosa in descending order of frequency

	%
Loss of appetite for carbohydrate foods	100
Loss of weight	99
Amenorrhoea*	91
Constipation	56
Feeling the cold	55
Fatigue	52
Insomnia	49
Abdominal discomfort	44
Nausea after eating	44
Giddiness	33
Headache	28
Nocturia	28
Vomiting after eating	21
Bulimic episodes	19
Dyspnoea on exertion	17

*Thirteen women were taking oral contraceptives.

denied that the appetite was otherwise affected. Twenty-nine patients (19%) described episodes of binging, and 33 (21%) confessed to self-induced vomiting, purgative abuse, or both. None of our patients were taking diuretics. The vomiters and purgers did not differ to any significant extent from the dieters with respect to their age, weight on presentation, or duration of weight loss.

No attempt was made to enquire too deeply about possible precipitating causes, but the patients were encouraged to talk freely to the medical and nursing staff. In two-thirds the condition appeared to have started during a period of emotional stress and these included concern over being overweight, worry about forthcoming examinations, difficulties with family or sexual relationships, and the death of a close relative. Psychological symptoms such as fear of fatness, overestimation of body size, and depression were frequently encountered.

Ten girls between 13 and 18 years of age and the patient with Turner's syndrome had primary amenorrhoea. One hundred and twenty-five females complained of secondary amenorrhoea and in 46% this had either preceded the beginning of the weight loss or had coincided with it. Regular monthly bleeding was still taking place in the 13 women on oral contraceptives and in some cases this had delayed referral. Two patients were postmenopausal. Other symptoms such as constipation, sensitivity to cold, fatigue and insomnia were particularly common (*Table 4.1*).

Physical findings

All the patients had clearly lost weight and one-third were described as emaciated. The most obvious feature was a marked loss of subcutaneous fat. Skin changes were commonplace and included lanugo, dryness, orange or yellow palms, and acrocyanosis. A slow pulse rate and hypotension were common. Half the patients had heart rates of less than 65 beats/minute, the slowest being 30 beats/minute. The lying systolic blood pressure was less than 100 mmHg in 43 patients. Secondary sexual characteristics tended to be well preserved, but atrophic breasts were recorded in 13

Table 4.2 Physical findings in 155 cases of anorexia nervosa in descending order of frequency

	%
Loss of subcutaneous fat	100
Lanugo	72
Dry skin	53
Bradycardia*	50
Emaciation	35
Hypotension†	29
Pallor	26
Orange-yellow palms	25
Acrocyanosis	21
Atrophic breasts	9
Scanty sexual hair	5
Ankle oedema	4

*Resting pulse rate less than 65 beats/minute.
† Supine systolic blood pressure of less than 100 mmHg.

long-standing cases (*Table 4.2*). Only one patient, who was grossly emaciated, was hypothermic; her rectal temperature on admission was 33.0°C.

Investigations

The haematological, biochemical and radiological abnormalities in these patients are described in the appropriate chapters and are only summarized here. All except a very few patients had normal haemoglobin levels on admission, but about one-third had white cell counts of less than 4.0×10^9/litre. Marrow biopsy in five cases with leucopenia showed the characteristic hypocellular marrow seen in this condition. Only three anorectics had evidence of platelet deficiency, and the erythrocyte sedimentation rate was normal in every case.

The serum electrolytes, creatinine and blood urea were normal in the majority of our patients, but hypokalaemia was present to some degree in 15 cases. Twenty-two had moderately elevated blood urea levels, but in only one instance was this associated with a raised serum creatinine level.

Liver function tests were abnormal in about one-third of our patients, the serum aspartate aminotransferase levels being most commonly affected. Normal serum calcium and phosphate concentrations were present in the majority, but one girl had undoubted biochemical evidence of osteomalacia which responded to vitamin D.

Routine chest radiographs failed to demonstrate any lung abnormalities but often revealed a small vertical heart which is characteristically seen in this condition.

Summary

The majority of our 155 cases were middle-class adolescent females whose illness was usually preceded by emotional stress and often accompanied by depression and an irrational fear of being overweight. The symptoms and signs were similar in prevalence to those described in other series, but there was an unexpectedly high incidence of fatigue. In addition, orange-yellow discoloration of the palms due to hypercarotenaemia was commoner than previously reported.

References

MATTINGLY, D. and BHANJI, S. (1982) The diagnosis of anorexia nervosa. *J. R. Coll. Physicians Lond.*, **16**, 191–194

RAMELL, M. D. and BROWN, N. (1988) Anorexia nervosa in a 67 year old lady. *Postgrad. Med. J.*, **64**, 48–49

TANNER, J. M. and WHITEHOUSE, R. H. (1975) *Growth and Development Record.* Castlemead: Castlemead Publications

Chapter 5

The cardiovascular system

From the earliest reports, those who encounter anorectics have been impressed by their seemingly boundless energy. Nevertheless, as was shown in the previous chapter, many anorectics do in fact complain of fatigue, dyspnoea or both. Examination usually reveals a slow pulse and a low blood pressure, and sometimes transient heart murmurs may be heard (Silverman, 1974). Oedema of the ankles is occasionally found, and may be difficult to explain, as it is seldom associated with cardiac failure or hypoproteinaemia. Indeed we have found raised serum albumin levels in many of our cases and this could not be explained by dehydration. Oedema may also be seen when the patients are beginning to gain weight, particularly if the patient is confined to bed (Maxmen, Siberfarb and Ferrell, 1974). This chapter is concerned with those special investigations which have been carried out on the cardiovascular system in patients with anorexia nervosa.

Peripheral circulation

Many anorectics complain of cold extremities, and acrocyanosis is a common finding. Freyschuss, Fohlin and Thoren (1978) investigated the peripheral circulation in 16 anorectics and 14 healthy controls, and found that calf blood flow was reduced by about half in the anorectics. The blood pressures in the arm and toes were also lower, as was the skin temperature measured at various levels below the knee. They suggested that selective peripheral vasoconstriction acts as a heat-conserving mechanism in these patients.

Heart size

In spite of the fact that since the early days of chest radiography there have been tables and charts relating heart size, as shown by the cardiac shadow on standard posteroanterior films, to body weight, it was widely believed that such a vital organ as the heart was spared in starvation. The work of Keys, Henschel and Taylor (1947) should have dispelled this view a long time ago. They carried out radiological measurements on 32 healthy young men who were subjected to semi-starvation for 6 months, during which time they lost one-quarter of their body weight. During this period the heart diminished in size and assumed a more vertical position. The heart

Table 5.1 Cardiothoracic ratios: comparison of patients and controls

	Patients	Controls	P (t test)
Mean age (years)	20.7	18.8	NS
Mean height (cm)	162.5	164.5	NS
Mean weight (kg)	37.4	58.8	<0.001
Mean weight (% optimum)	67.3	102.7	<0.001
Mean cardiothoracic ratio (%)	36.9	42.2	<0.001

NS: not significant

shadow enlarged when the diet was increased, but did not resume its former appearance until a free choice of food was permitted.

It has been known for some time that a small vertical heart is a characteristic feature of Addison's disease. Heymsfield *et al.* (1978) have shown that a narrow cardiac shadow may also be seen in patients with other physical illnesses which result in weight loss. Their 10 patients included three with malignant disease. Three more were suffering from Crohn's disease, cirrhosis and peptic ulceration respectively, and two had received abdominal surgery which had resulted in malabsorption.

Relatively little interest has been shown in the size of the heart in anorexia nervosa as measured by the cardiothoracic ratio. Where the chest radiograph has been mentioned there is usually no comment on the heart. Thus, Kanis *et al.* (1974) reported no abnormal findings, and Beck and Brochner-Mortensen (1954) and Haller *et al.* (1977) stated that only infrequently was the cardiac shadow small. By contrast, Moodie and Salcedo (1983) found that 10 of their 12 anorectics had cardiothoracic ratios of less than 40%, the lowest value being 32%. We have confirmed their finding in our own patients. The chest radiographs of 35 female anorectics with a weight loss of at least 20% of their calculated optimum weight were compared with those of an equal number of healthy subjects. The latter consisted of female students who had a chest X-ray taken as part of a routine medical examination. The cardiothoracic ratio was measured from standard-size posteroanterior chest films (Sutton, 1980).

Although the mean age and height of the patients were similar to those of the controls, their mean weight and cardiothoracic ratio were lower (*Table 5.1*). No statistically significant correlation could be demonstrated between the anorectics' heart size and their weight. The mean cardiothoracic ratio of those anorectics who had been ill for less than 2 years (36.0%) was significantly lower ($P<0.05$) than that of the more chronic anorectics (38.8%). The mean cardiothoracic ratio in those with bradycardia (34.7%) was lower ($P<0.01$) than in those with higher pulse rates (38.7%).

Eleven patients were reassessed after successful treatment; their mean cardiothoracic ratio had increased from 35.5% to 42.8%, a value close to that in the controls. This change was statistically significant ($P<0.01$). In every instance the increase in the transverse cardiac diameter exceeded that usually seen between systole and diastole (Simon, 1968). A typical example is shown in *Figure 5.1*.

It is possible that the small heart shadow merely reflects loss of cardiac fat which we have seen at autopsy. On the other hand, echocardiographic studies have suggested that it may be due to a reduction in left ventricular mass (Gottdiener *et al.*, 1978; Moodie and Salcedo, 1983). Reduced blood volume may also play a part (Fohlin *et al.*, 1978). If this were so, it would provide a common link with Addison's disease, the only other condition in which a reduced cardiothoracic ratio is frequently found.

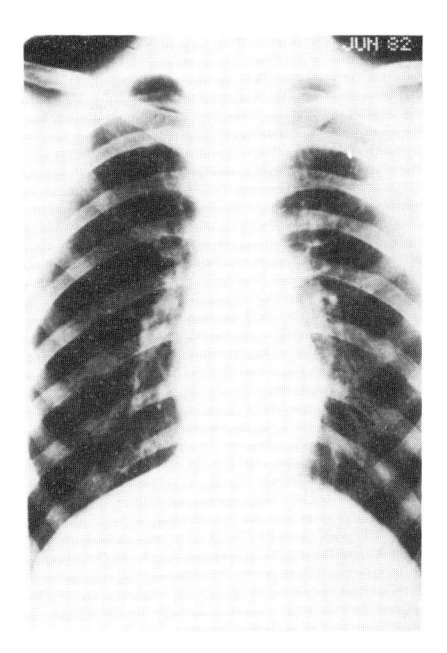

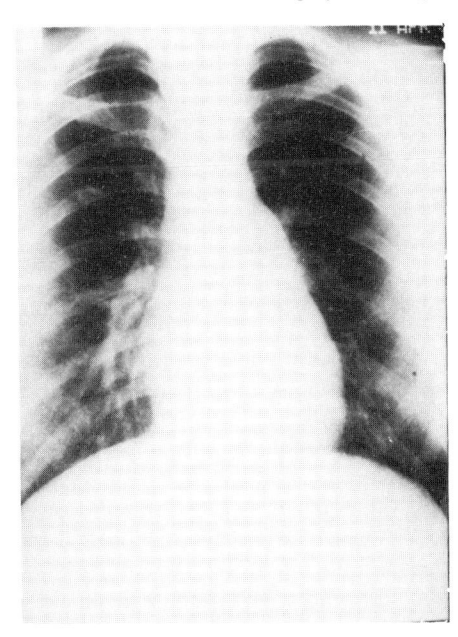

Figure 5.1 (Left) Chest X-ray to show small vertical heart in a 14-year-old girl before treatment. (Right) Repeat chest X-ray 10 months later when fully recovered. The cardiothoracic ratio is now normal

Electrocardiographic findings

Sudden death in anorexia nervosa may be due to cardiac arrhythmias. The electrocardiograph (ECG) has been investigated in semi-starved healthy volunteers, patients with organic wasting diseases, and in anorectics. Simonson, Henschel and Keys (1947) reported a number of ECG changes in young men whose diet had been severely restricted for 24 weeks: bradycardia occurred, the QT interval increased, there was an overall decrease in amplitude, and the QRS and T axes shifted to the right. By contrast, Heymsfield et al. (1978) found normal ECGs in those who had lost weight because of various physical illnesses.

A variety of ECG changes have been observed in anorectics, the commonest being a sinus bradycardia. One of the earliest reports of this was by Berkman (1930), who described a severely emaciated youth with a heart rate of only 44 beats/minute. There were no other ECG abnormalities. Beck and Brochner-Mortensen (1954) also found a bradycardia in seven of their 18 patients. More recent reports of sinus bradycardia include those of Warren and Vande Wiele (1973), Silverman (1974) and Palossy and Oo (1977). Brotman and Stern (1983) reported one of the slowest heart rates. The patient was a cachetic 25-year-old woman who, although alert, was so weak as to be barely able to walk. An ECG confirmed a bradycardia of only 25 heart beats each minute, but showed no other abnormality. As the patient's weight increased, so did her pulse rate. Mitchell and Gillum (1980) described an irregular bradycardia in a 25-year-old anorectic whose serum electrolytes, including magnesium, were within normal limits. Her ECG showed sinus rhythm with frequent supraventricular premature beats and an abnormal P wave axis. This, together with a PR interval of 0.12 s, suggested a junctional focus with retrograde atrial conduction. During the course of weight gain, achieved by behaviour therapy, the ECG became normal. In the same year Gould et al. (1980) investigated a 30-year-old anorectic who presented with syncopal attacks. The ECG on admission showed a sinus bradycardia, but no other changes. His bundle electrocardiography, however, revealed a conduction defect. This resolved spontaneously as weight was regained. We have come across a grossly emaciated 18-year-old anorectic who, on admission to hospital, was found to have a pulse rate of only 30 beats/minute. An ECG showed intermittent first and second degree heart block, but this became normal as she gained weight. This had not been previously reported in anorexia nervosa, but intermittent Wenkebach type second degree block commonly occurs at night in normal children and adolescents and is thought to be a vagal effect. In the anorectic described by Gould et al. (1980) atropine resulted in a marked increase in the pulse rate. It seems reasonable to assume that the bradycardia in this disorder may be due to vagal overactivity.

As well as changes in heart rate, alterations in the configuration of the ECG have also been reported. Silverman (1974) found non-specific changes in most of his anorectics; these were more marked in those with the greatest weight losses and included generalized low voltage and reduced or inverted T waves. In none of his cases was there any disturbance of acid-base balance or plasma electrolyte levels.

Thurston and Marks (1974) studied nine anorectics aged between 13 and 19 years and two older patients with comparable degrees of weight loss, but due to depression and schizophrenia respectively. The ECGs of the anorectics showed a variety of abnormalities. These included the frequent presence of T-wave inversion or flattening, together with ST depression and minor prolongation of the QT interval in five cases. There were no electrolyte disturbances at the time. The authors contrasted the many changes seen in the anorectics with the normal ECGs seen in the two other patients, and suggested that there are ECG abnormalities which are specific to anorexia nervosa. They postulated that these were due to the release of catecholamines within the myocardium, and that this in turn was due to overstimulation of hypothalamic sympathetic centres.

The opinion that the ECG changes in anorexia nervosa arise from the central nervous system was shared by Palossy and Oo (1977). The ECGs of 10 of their 16 patients showed either sinus tachycardia or bradycardia. T waves were usually flat or inverted, ST depression was a common finding, and U waves were seen in seven cases. Warren and Steinberg (1979) mentioned two hypokalaemic anorectics with U waves in their discussion of the potential consequences of blood electrolyte disturbances in anorexia nervosa, and regarded these as of more significance than a hypothetical hypothalamic disorder. A third possible explanation for the abnormal ECG in this condition is myocardial damage as a result of severe starvation (Garnett et al., 1969).

There is little evidence that the ECG changes described above have any effect on the prognosis, with the possible exception of the presence of U waves due to hypokalaemia, or a prolonged QT interval. Isner et al. (1985) recently reported three fatal cases, for whom no obvious cause of death could be found at autopsy. During the week before death they all showed prolongation of the QT interval. Corrected for heart rate, the values were 0.61, 0.47 and 0.46 s respectively. Terminal ECGs showed ventricular tachycardia followed by cardiac arrest.

Myocardial efficiency

A low blood pressure is a common feature of anorexia nervosa, and inevitably raises the question as to whether there is a reduction in myocardial efficiency. There are, however, conflicting views on this. Fohlin *et al.* (1978) reported that the left ventricular stroke volume was well maintained, and this has been confirmed by others (Gottdiener *et al.*, 1978; Moodie and Salcedo, 1983; St John Sutton *et al.*, 1985). On the other hand, Kalager, Brubakk and Bassoe (1978) and Murphy *et al.* (1985) found impaired myocardial activity in their cases.

Mitral valve prolapse

Oka *et al.* (1984) using echocardiography observed this abnormality in 14 of their 19 anorectics. They did not find any differences in left ventricular size, mass or performance between those cases with mitral valve prolapse and those without, but the former had lower pulse rates. Johnson *et al.* (1986) also found mitral valve prolapse in half their cases and suggested that changes in thoracic cage configuration could be responsible. By contrast, Meyers *et al.* (1986), who detected mitral valve prolapse in only one-third of their patients, felt that reduced left ventricle size was at least a contributory factor. Whatever the causes in anorexia nervosa, it would appear to be an asymptomatic finding which is revealed only by auscultation or echocardiography. Unfortunately the criteria used in diagnosing mitral valve prolapse are variable, so that incidence studies between different observers may give inconsistent findings.

Ipecac cardiotoxicity

Anorectics who habitually vomit place their hearts at risk through hypokalaemia. Another less well-recognized hazard is the use of ipecac syrup which, in the UK, the USA and Canada, is available without prescription. The main active constituents of this emetic are the alkaloids emetine and cephalin. The latter causes greater nausea and vomiting, but emetine is more cardiotoxic. Adler *et al.* (1980) have described an anorectic who died after drinking 90–100 ml of ipecac syrup daily for 3 months. She presented with complaints of palpitations, tightness of the chest, dyspnoea on exertion, and fatigue. On examination, even slight movement resulted in breathlessness: she had a regular tachycardia of 150 beats/minute, was hypotensive (75/60 mmHg), and a summation gallop was heard over the precordium. The chest radiograph was reported as normal, but the ECG showed a supraventricular tachycardia and inverted T waves. In spite of intensive medical care the patient died in ventricular fibrillation. Friedman (1984) has described the autopsy findings in an anorectic who succumbed to the affects of ipecac. The myocardium showed inflammatory changes and degeneration of its fibres; a fibrous pericarditis was also present. In addition, marked myopathic and degenerative changes were seen in the skeletal muscles.

Although their findings apply to North American cases of bulimia nervosa, some idea of the extent of ipecac abuse can be gleaned from the report by Pope *et al.* (1986). This suggested that approximately a quarter of a million American women use this preparation to control their weight. At the time of writing there is a strong lobby in North America for making ipecac syrup a prescription-only drug. As yet ipecac abuse does not appear to be a major problem in the UK.

Other cardiac complications

Cardiovascular problems may arise in the course of treatment. In their paper describing an anorectic with profound bradycardia, Mitchell and Gillum (1980) emphasized that, even where there is no evident metabolic abnormality, patients should be carefully assessed if treatment with a potentially cardiotoxic drug, such as a tricyclic antidepressant, is contemplated. However, Powers (1982) has pointed out that cardiac problems can occur in patients who are not receiving any medication. She described three cases who had been admitted to psychiatric wards for behaviour therapy. At varying intervals after weight gain had commenced each one developed a tachycardia and signs of heart failure. Although the causes were obscure it was discovered that one patient persuaded her parents to bring in high-salt foods.

Fonseca and Havard (1985) have stressed the need for regular biochemical review. They reported on a 32-year-old chronic laxative and diuretic abuser who was emaciated on admission, but had no signs of heart failure. Her anaemia responded to a blood transfusion, but potassium and calcium supplements had no appreciable effect on her hypokalaemia or hypocalcaemia. A week after her admission, the patient developed symptoms and signs of congestive cardiac failure. This responded poorly to treatment, and further investigations were carried out. The patient was found to be hypomagnesaemic and was given an infusion of magnesium sulphate. The serum potassium and calcium levels soon became normal and the heart failure rapidly resolved.

Summary

The commonest cardiovascular abnormalities in this disease are acrocyanosis, bradycardia, hypotension and decreased heart size. Since similar changes are seen in starvation they are probably a consequence of the nutritional state of the patient. Most of the cardiovascular complications are benign, but in some patients there is a risk of sudden death from cardiac arrhythmias.

References

ADLER, A. F., WALINSKY, P., KRALL, R. A. and CHO, S. Y. (1980) Death resulting from ipecac syrup poisoning. *J. Am. Med. Assoc.*, **243**, 1927–1928

BECK, J. C. and BROCHNER-MORTENSEN, K. (1954) Observations on the prognosis in anorexia nervosa. *Acta Med. Scand.*, **149**, 409–430

BERKMAN, J. M. (1930) Anorexia nervosa, anorexia, inanation, and low basal metabolic rate. *Am. J. Med. Sci.*, **180**, 411–424

BROTMAN, A. W. and STERN, T. A. (1983) Case report of cardiovascular abnormalities in anorexia nervosa. *Am. J. Psychiatry*, **140**, 1227–1228

FOHLIN, L., FREYSCHUSS, U., BJARKE, B., DAVIES, C. T. M. and THOREN, C. (1978) Function and dimensions of the circulatory system in anorexia nervosa. *Acta Paediatr. Scand.*, **67**, 11–16

FONSECA, V. and HAVARD, C. W. H. (1985) Electrolyte disturbances and cardiac failure with hypomagnesaemia in anorexia nervosa. *Br. Med. J.*, **291**, 1680–1682

FREYSCHUSS, U., FOHLIN, L. and THOREN, C. (1978) Limb circulation in anorexia nervosa. *Acta Paediatr. Scand.*, **67**, 225–228

FRIEDMAN, E. J. (1984) Death from ipecac intoxication in a patient with anorexia nervosa. *Am. J. Psychiatry*, **141**, 702–703

GARNETT, E. S., BARNARD, D. L., FORD, J. GOODBODY, R. A. and WOODEHOUSE, M. A. (1969) Gross fragmentation of cardiac myofibrils after therapeutic starvation for obesity. *Lancet*, i, 914–916

GOTTDIENER, J. S., GROSS, H. A., HENRY, W. L., BORER, J. S. and EBERT, M. H. (1978) Effects of self-induced starvation on cardiac size and function in anorexia nervosa. *Circulation*, **58**, 425–433

GOULD, L., REDDY, C. V. R., SINGH, B. K. and ZEN, B. (1980) Evaluation of cardiac conduction in anorexia nervosa. *P.A.C.E.*, **3**, 660–665

HALLER, J. O., SLOVIS, T. L., BAKER, D. H., BERDON, W. E. and SILVERMAN, J. A. (1977) Anorexia nervosa—the paucity of radiological findings in more than fifty patients. *Pediatr. Radiol.*, **5**, 145–147

HEYMSFIELD, S. B., BETHEL, R. A., ANSLEY, J. D., GIBBS, D. M., FELNER, J. M. and NUTTER, D. O. (1978) Cardiac abnormalities in cachectic patients before and during nutritional repletion. *Am. Heart J.*, **95**, 584–594

ISNER, J. M., ROBERTS, W. C., HEYMSFIELD, S. B. and YAGER, J. (1985) Anorexia nervosa and sudden death. *Ann. Intern. Med.*, **102**, 49–52

JOHNSON, G. L., HUMPHRIES, L. L., SHIRLEY, P. B., MAZZOLENI, A. and NOONAN, J. A. (1986) Mitral valve prolapse in patients with anorexia nervosa and bulimia. *Arch. Int. Med.*, **146**, 1525–1529

KALAGER, T., BRUBAKK, O. and BASSOE, H. H. (1978) Cardiac performance in patients with anorexia nervosa. *Cardiology*, **63**, 1–4

KANIS, J. A., BROWN, P., FITZPATRICK, K., HIBBERT, D. J., HORN, D. B., NAIRN, I. M. et al. (1974) Anorexia nervosa: a clinical, psychiatric and laboratory study. *Q. J. Med.*, **67**, 321–328

KEYS, A., HENSCHEL, A. and TAYLOR, H. L. (1947) The size and function of the human heart at rest in semi-starvation and in subsequent rehabilitation. *Am. J. Physiol.*, **150**, 153–169

MAXMEN, J. S., SIBERFARB, P. M. and FERRELL, R. B. (1974) Anorexia nervosa: practical initial management in a general hospital. *J. Am. Med. Assoc.*, **229**, 801–803

MEYERS, D. G., STARKE, H., PEARSON, P. H. and WILKEN, M. K. (1986) Mitral valve prolapse in anorexia nervosa. *Ann. Int. Med.*, **105**, 384–386

MITCHELL, J. E. and GILLUM, R. (1980) Weight-dependent arrhythmia in a patient with anorexia nervosa. *Am. J. Psychiatry*, **137**, 377–378

MOODIE, D. S. and SALCEDO, E. (1983) Cardiac function in adolescents and young adults with anorexia nervosa. *J. Adolesc. Health Care*, **4**, 9–14

MURPHY, D. J., DICKSON, T. M, BRUNNER, R. L., MALONEY, M. J., FARRELL, M. K., MEYER, R. A. et al. (1985) Concomitant psychological improvement during successful treatment of anorexia nervosa. *J. Adolesc. Health Care*, **6**, 392–396

OKA, Y., ITO, T., SEKINE, I., SADA, T., OKABE, F., NAITO, A. et al. (1984) Mitral valve prolapse in patients with anorexia nervosa. *J. Cardiogr.*, **14**, 483–491

PALOSSY, B. and OO, M. (1977) ECG alteration in anorexia nervosa. *Adv. Cardiol.*, **19**, 280–282

POPE, H. G., HUDSON, J. I., NIXON, R. A. and HERRIDGE, P. L. (1986) The epidemiology of ipecac abuse. *N. Eng. J. Med.*, **314**, 245–246

POWERS, P. S. (1982) Heart failure during treatment of anorexia nervosa. *Am. J. Psychiatry*, **139**, 1167–1170

ST JOHN SUTTON, M. G., PLAPPERT, T., CROSBY, L., DOUGLAS, P., MULLEN, J. and REICHEK, N. (1985) Effects of reduced left ventricular mass on chamber architecture, load, and function: a study of anorexia nervosa. *Circulation*, **72**, 991–1000

SILVERMAN, J. A. (1974) Anorexia nervosa: clinical observations in a successful treatment plan. *J. Pediatr.*, **84**, 68–73

SIMON, G. (1968) The limitations of the radiograph for detecting heart enlargement. *Br. J. Radiol.*, **41**, 862–865

SIMONSON, E., HENSCHEL, A. and KEYS, A. (1947) The electrocardiogram of man in semistarvation and subsequent rehabilitation. *Am. Heart J.*, **35**, 584–602

SUTTON, D. (1980) *A Textbook of Radiology and Imagery*. Edinburgh: Churchill Livingstone

THURSTON, J. and MARKS, P. (1974) Electrocardiographic abnormalities in patients with anorexia nervosa. *Br. Heart J.*, **36**, 719–723

WARREN, M. P. and VANDE WIELE, R. L. (1973) Clinical and metabolic features of anorexia nervosa. *Am. J. Obstet. Gynecol.*, **117**, 435–449

WARREN, S. E. and STEINBERG, S. M. (1979) Acid-base and electrolyte disturbances in anorexia nervosa. *Am. J. Psychiatry*, **136**, 415–418

Chapter 6

The respiratory system

In the past pneumonia, often tubercular in origin, was a frequent terminal event in anorexia nervosa (Ryle, 1936). Fortunately respiratory complications are now relatively rare and easily treated. Only five of our patients, all grossly emaciated, developed chest infections after admission to hospital. Four had pneumonia and one was found to have a lung abscess. All these infections resolved with antibiotics and physiotherapy. Anorectics who vomit regularly are at greater risk as vomitus may be inhaled. Warren and Vande Wiele (1973) described a patient with an aperistaltic oesophagus in whom an aspiration pneumonia may have contributed to death. One of the cases described by Gryboski et al. (1980) and who developed pancreatitis had a grossly distended stomach, and inhalation of some of its contents may have led to her pneumonia.

A spontaneous pneumothorax occurred in a case described by Crisp and Stonehill (1967). The patient concerned would periodically go on carbohydrate binges which would end only when she felt dizzy, short of breath, and bloated. The pneumothorax happened at the end of a binge which had gone on for 2 weeks and had resulted in a gain of some 25 kg! Pneumothorax has also been reported as a complication in an anorectic nourished via a catheter in the superior vena cava (Pertschuk et al., 1981).

Pneumomediastinum, an unusual complication, was first described by Al-Mufty and Bevan (1977). A 16-year-old grossly underweight anorectic was admitted and placed on the normal hospital diet. Each meal was followed by discomfort, but on the second day she developed upper abdominal pain. Examination revealed epigastric tenderness and widespread surgical emphysema over the lower part of the neck, the thorax and the abdomen. Radiological examination showed mediastinal, retroperitoneal and subcutaneous adventitious air. Other investigations revealed nothing untoward apart from a raised blood urea and a polymorph leucocytosis. Gastrografin studies, barium meal, barium enema and laparotomy all failed to demonstrate any gastrointestinal or peritoneal pathology. As the patient was never observed to vomit or hyperventilate, the authors suggested that the air leakage occurred as the result of inanition weakening the connective tissue of the lungs.

Two further cases were reported by Donley and Kemple (1978). Both were young girls, and the second was known deliberately to vomit. In the first, a chest radiograph 24 hours after admission showed pneumomediastinum and pneumopericardium; later, surgical emphysema developed in the neck. Barium studies revealed no abnormality. The patient remained asymptomatic, and within a few days the emphysema had disappeared and the chest radiograph was normal. The second case was similar, but the presence of surgical emphysema was noted on admission and the chest radiograph showed mediastinal emphysema only. The authors noted that the lungs of starved rats show an increase in alveolar surface forces and a decrease in tissue elasticity, and suggested that comparable changes could occur in anorexia nervosa. Another example was that of Brooks and Martin (1979), who believed that in their case of pneumomediastinum vomiting was the most probable precipitating factor.

The patient reported by Altmeyer and Morgan (1981) is of particular interest as a spontaneous pneumomediastinum was the presenting feature. A 19-year-old girl sought medical attention after waking with mild pleuritic substernal pain which radiated to the right shoulder. Being concerned that she had glandular fever, she felt her neck for enlarged lymph nodes and found it to be swollen and noticed a crackling sensation. Physical examination revealed a cachectic young girl with pharyngeal inflammation and widespread surgical emphysema in the neck; auscultation disclosed a crunching sound over the heart which was synchronous with its beats. A chest radiograph showed a pneumomediastinum with air around the pericardium, and confirmed the presence of subcutaneous air in the neck. The chest pain disappeared within 48 hours, and the subcutaneous emphysema within a week. She was subsequently seen by a psychiatrist who confirmed the diagnosis of anorexia nervosa.

The most recent example is the anorectic reported by Fergusson, Shaw and Turnbull (1985). This patient had been ill for 3 years when she developed retrosternal pain radiating to the back and left shoulder. As with most of the other cases, there was no history of vomiting. Supraclavicular surgical emphysema was present, as was a praecordial rasp in time with the heart beat. There was marked sinus bradycardia (22 beats/minute) and hypotension (80/50 mmHg). Radiography revealed air in the neck, and showed that air in the mediastinum had tracked downwards into the abdominal cavity through the aortic opening in the diaphragm.

Only one of our patients has ever developed surgical emphysema in the neck. It was asymptomatic and was first discovered on a chest radiograph which was otherwise normal. She denied self-induced vomiting, but later developed a lung abscess which could have been due to aspiration.

Summary

In our experience respiratory infections are rare and amenable to treatment. The risk of aspiration pneumonia is greatest in those who indulge in self-induced vomiting, but this habit is rarely associated with leakage of air from the lungs into the pleural cavity or adjacent tissues.

References

AL-MUFTY, N. S. and BEVAN, D. H. (1977) A case of subcutaneous emphysema, pneumomediastinum and pneumoperitoneum associated with functional anorexia. *Br. J. Clin. Pract.*, **31**, 160–161

ALTMEYER, R. B. and MORGAN, E. J. (1981) Spontaneous pneumomediastinum as a complication of anorexia nervosa. *W. Va. Med. J.*, **77**, 189–190

BROOKS, A. P. and MARTIN, C. (1979) Pneumomediastinum in anorexia nervosa. *Br. Med. J.*, i, 124

CRISP, A. H. and STONEHILL, E. (1967) Hypercarotenaemia as a symptom of weight phobia. *Postgrad. Med. J.*, **43**, 721–725

DONLEY, A. J. and KEMPLE, T. J. (1978) Spontaneous pneumomediastinum complicating anorexia nervosa. *Br. Med. J.*, ii, 1604–1605

FERGUSSON, R. J., SHAW, T. R. D. and TURNBULL, C. M. (1985) Spontaneous pneumomediastinum: a complication of anorexia nervosa? *Postgrad. Med. J.*, **61**, 815–817

GRYBOSKI, J., HILLMEIER, C., KOCOSHIS, S., ANYAN, W. and SEASHORE, J. S. (1980) Refeeding pancreatitis in malnourished children. *J. Pediatr.*, **97**, 441–443

PERTSCHUK, M. J., FORSTER, J., BUZBY, G. and MULLEN, J. L. (1981) The treatment of anorexia nervosa with total parenteral nutrition. *Biol. Psychiatry*, **16**, 539–550

RYLE, J. A. (1936) Anorexia nervosa. *Lancet*, ii, 893–899

WARREN, M. P. and VANDE WIELE, R. L. (1973) Clinical and metabolic features of anorexia nervosa. *Am. J. Obstet. Gynecol.*, **117**, 435–449

Chapter 7

The nervous system

Epilepsy is the most striking neurological abnormality seen in patients with anorexia nervosa, and occurs in a significant proportion of cases. It may be a consequence of the disease itself or a side-effect of treatment. Dally and Sargant (1966) reported an incidence of 17% of convulsions in their patients within a fortnight of starting treatment with chlorpromazine and insulin. Chlorpromazine lowers the epileptic threshold and the dosage of insulin was sufficient to cause hypoglycaemia in grossly emaciated patients. We ourselves have unwittingly produced severe hypoglycaemia and consequent convulsions in two of our patients following a dose of only two units of insulin subcutaneously. In a small number of cases there is a history of idiopathic epilepsy or evidence of previous brain damage. Other neurological complications have been reported but may not be complained of by the patient. They are more likely to be detected during clinical examination or by special investigations such as electroencephalography and computed tomography of the brain.

Neuropsychology

It is widely believed that anorectics are of average or above average intelligence. Nevertheless, some investigators have demonstrated defects in higher cerebral functioning in some of their cases.

Hamsher, Halmi and Benton (1981) found a number of cognitive defects in their 20 patients. The commonest were retarded reaction time, defective short-term visual memory and impaired information retrieval. These were unrelated to a history of birth complications, depression, bulimia, vomiting or purgative abuse. Those in whom cognitive defects were still present after refeeding tended to have lower weights when reviewed one year later. The authors suggested that there may be some anorectics in whom an organic disorder of the central nervous system limits their capacity for recovery.

Further evidence of cognitive abnormalities has been provided by Fox (1981–82) who proposed that anorexia nervosa may be associated with right hemisphere dysfunction, and by Strupp et al. (1986) who favoured a central neurochemical disturbance. However, Gordon, Halmi and Ippolito (1984) found no consistent pattern of cognitive impairment in their cases. They did, nevertheless, observe that the anorectics' learning strategies resembled those used by young children.

The significance of the above findings is still uncertain. They may result from unrecognized brain damage in infancy which predisposes toward anorexia nervosa

(Halmi, 1974; Artmann et al., 1985). Alternatively they may represent transient consequences of the illness or its treatment (Kohlmeyer, Lehmkuhl and Poutska, 1983).

Electroencephalography

There have been a number of studies of the electroencephalogram (EEG) in untreated anorectics, but the majority of these have involved only a few patients and lack clinical detail. Two notable exceptions are the reports of Crisp, Fenton and Scotton (1968) and Nell et al. (1980).

An early study, involving only three patients, demonstrated irregular mixtures of low to moderate activity of 12–16 cycles/s (DuBois, 1949). Goor (1954) had three patients with EEG changes which the author regarded as indicating brainstem dysfunction. He further suggested that this abnormality might be congenital in origin, as 11 out of 15 relatives had similar EEGs. Martin (1955) described the appearances of the brains of two anorectics at autopsy and found them to be similar to those seen in pellagra. He suggested that similar changes could have accounted for the abnormal EEGs in two other cases. One had an unusually slow dominant rhythm, the other a diffuse dysrhythmia, and both reacted abnormally to photic stimulation.

Heidrich and Schmidt-Matthias (1961), in a paper concerned more with air encephalography, mentioned two patients with dysrhythmic EEGs. Seven anorectics were reported by Gibbs and Gibbs (1964). They all had normal recordings, apart from two who had been treated with ACTH. Dally and Sargant (1966) reported an incidence of 25% of abnormal EEGs in their untreated cases. Similar non-specific changes have been recorded by others (Lundberg and Walinder, 1967; Shimoda and Kitagawa, 1973; Kanis et al., 1974; Kohlmeyer, Lehmkuhl and Poutska, 1983; Grebb, Yingling and Reus, 1984). Suematsu et al. (1985) collected data on over 1000 Japanese cases. They divided their subjects into typical anorectics who fulfilled strict diagnostic criteria, and atypical ones where the criteria were less stringent. The EEG abnormalities were not specified, but were commoner among the typical cases (39%) than among the rest (22%). By contrast, Silverman (1974) found no EEG abnormalities in his 29 patients.

The first comprehensive account of the EEG in anorexia nervosa was by Crisp, Fenton and Scotton (1968). They investigated 32 anorectics before they had started treatment and the same number of sex and age-matched healthy volunteers of normal weight. Abnormal background activity, defined as slowing of the dominant frequency, occurred in 59% of the patients, but in only 22% of the controls. The four patients with bilaterally synchronous 4–6/s spike and wave complexes all had a history of convulsions. The response to hyperventilation was unstable in 31% of the anorectics as opposed to 9% of the healthy subjects. The major influence on the EEG was the duration of the illness, those ill for more than 5 years having a higher proportion of abnormalities. Abnormal EEGs were more common in the presence of low sodium, potassium or chloride levels. Two severely hypothermic patients had marked slowing of the dominant activity. The EEG did not appear to be affected by the patient's weight, nor did it bear any relationship to the response to treatment.

Nell et al. (1980) investigated 36 patients with primary anorexia nervosa of whom nearly half had abnormal EEGs. The commonest finding was of generalized slowing of background activity, but some had spike and wave complexes. Age and the extent of weight loss had no effect on the EEG, and contrary to the finding of Crisp, Fenton and Scotton (1968) neither did the duration of weight loss. The pure dieters usually had a normal EEG. The 12 patients who had a metabolic alkalosis were evenly distributed between those with normal EEGs and those with abnormal records.

From this brief review it is apparent that non-specific abnormalities in the EEG in anorectic patients are not uncommon. The most frequent finding is of generalized slow wave activity. Where fits have occurred the EEG is likely to show spike and wave complexes. Whether these changes are due to starvation, primary brain damage, or some obscure metabolic disturbance is uncertain.

Neuroradiology

Standard skull radiographs should not be requested routinely for they rarely show any abnormality and are not usually indicated (Kanis et al., 1974; Haller et al., 1977). There is no convincing evidence that the pituitary fossa is reduced in size (Bergstrom, Lundberg and Sjovall, 1973).

Because of their unpleasant nature, carotid angiography or air encephalography have been carried out on only a few patients. Lundberg and Walinder (1967) reported that bilateral carotid angiograms revealed nothing untoward in an anorectic with pre-existing epilepsy, but air encephalography in another showed a dilated left lateral ventricle. Geisler (1953) and Heidrich and Schmidt-Matthias (1961) also demonstrated ventricular dilatation, accompanied by widening of the cortical sulci, in anorectics who had lost considerable amounts of weight.

With the advent of non-invasive neuroradiological techniques it has been possible to investigate a larger number of patients. The first reports that computed tomography revealed cerebral atrophy in some cases of anorexia nervosa appeared in 1977. Enzmann and Lane (1977) studied four patients of whom three had bilateral, symmetrical widening of the cortical sulci. There was no evidence of dehydration, hypoalbuminaemia or electrolyte disturbance to account for this, but one patient had an abnormal EEG. Heinz, Martinez and Haenggeli (1977) found more extensive changes, in that widening of the sulci was accompanied by ventricular dilatation. After weight restoration the appearance of the brain became normal.

Nussbaum et al. (1980) reported their findings in 14 cases. Half the subjects had ventricular enlargement, wide sulci or both. These abnormalities were reported as commoner in male cases, and in those with a greater extent and rate of weight loss. In the two patients who were reassessed after weight gain, the abnormalities had persisted, albeit to a lesser extent in one. Sauer, Hornstein and Kessler (1985) have also described a case in which cerebral atrophy persisted after successful treatment. On the other hand, Zeumer, Hacke and Hartwich (1982) reported two cases in whom the atrophic appearances were reversed after weight gain.

Similar reports of cerebral atrophy have been provided by Luton et al. (1981), Suematsu et al. (1985) and Datlof et al. (1986). Cerebellar atrophy has been observed by Cala and Mastaglia (1980) in two out of four anorectics, and by Sein et al. (1981) in a 14-year-old prepubertal anorectic with substantial loss of weight and an abnormal EEG. After successful treatment, the radiological and EEG findings returned to normal. Further accounts of cerebellar atrophy include those of Berant, Mandel and Goldsher (1984) and Emrich et al. (1984).

Kohlmeyer, Lehmkuhl and Poutska (1983) studied 23 patients of whom 21 had markedly dilated cortical sulci and abnormal EEGs. They found that the cerebral atrophy was accompanied by impaired concentration, reaction time and perceptual

40 The nervous system

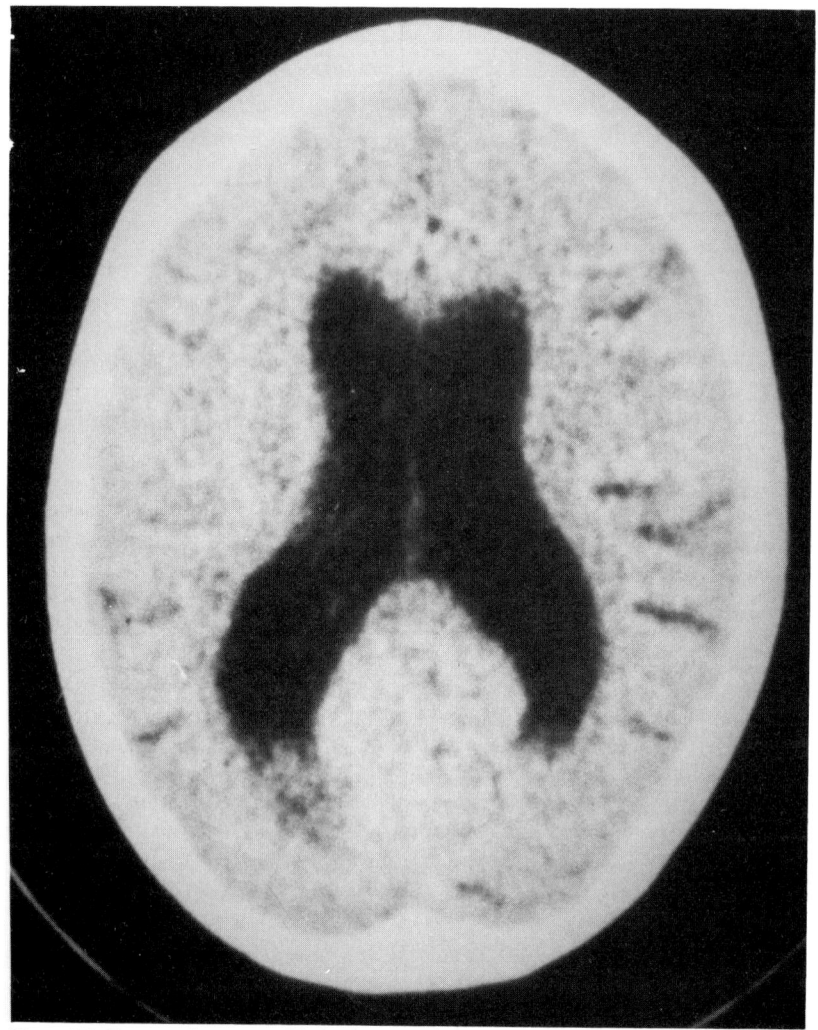

Figure 7.1 Computed tomographic brain scan of a 14-year-old girl with severe anorexia nervosa showing grossly dilated ventricles and widened sulci

speed, but not by diminished overall intelligence. Lankenau et al. (1985) also found no correlation between cerebral atrophy and intelligence.

The highest incidence of abnormalities is that reported by Artmann et al. (1985) who investigated 35 anorectics. Cortical changes occurred in 32 (91%), ventricular enlargement in 27 (77%), and cerebellar changes in 17 (49%). There was no correlation between the brain appearances and the length of the illness. EEG recordings were carried out in 29 subjects, and were abnormal in 12. Brain scans were repeated in 26 patients after weight gain and showed some improvement which was more marked in those who had put on the most weight. Nevertheless, in 31% the ventricles remained enlarged, and the authors thought that this was evidence for pre-existing brain damage acquired early in life. A number of these cases had a history of premature birth, difficult delivery or retarded early development.

We have investigated the brain scans in 29 unselected female patients admitted with eating disorders. Twenty-three of these had anorexia nervosa and six had bulimia nervosa. The mean age of the anorectics was 18.1 years, but the bulimics were older, their mean age being 25.3 years. An abnormal scan was found in only one of the bulimics, who had dilated lateral ventricles. By contrast, six of the anorectics had widened sulci, one had dilated lateral ventricles, and three had both abnormalities (*Figure 7.1*). The mean serum albumin level in these 10 patients was lower than that found in those anorectics with 'normal' brains (41.5 g/l *versus* 48.1 g/l; $P<0.02$). No statistically significant differences could be demonstrated with respect to age, duration and extent of weight loss, self-induced vomiting or purging, short-term response to treatment, pulse rate, systolic blood pressure, serum electrolytes, and haemoglobin level. Krieg, Backmund and Pirke (1987) have also shown that cerebral atrophy may be observed in cases of bulimia nervosa and have therefore commented that weight loss alone cannot be held responsible.

With the increasing use of computed tomography of the brain it is becoming clear that evidence of cerebral atrophy is not uncommon in anorexia nervosa. There is still uncertainty as to whether it resolves completely or whether it has any effect on prognosis. What is certain is that it may take several months after refeeding before the appearances return to normal. Despite these structural abnormalities, Emrich *et al.* (1984), using positron emission tomography, found no evidence of abnormal brain glucose metabolism.

Neuromuscular disorders

Muscle weakness, when it occurs in anorexia nervosa, is often attributed to potassium depletion. This is usually associated with an inadequate intake, excessive vomiting, or purgative abuse. Nightingale, Smith and Turnbull (1981) reported another cause which was not immediately apparent. A 25-year-old woman was admitted with painful and weak proximal muscles following an influenza-like illness 3 months previously. For about one month she had been troubled by polyuria and nocturia, and had been noted to be hypokalaemic. Oral potassium had been prescribed and the patient had taken no other medication. Her weight had been stable for 5 years at some 20 g below the optimum for her age and height. Her limbs were thin, but the tendon reflexes were normal and sensation was intact. Her blood pressure was 110/70 mmHg. Investigation showed a hypokalaemic alkalosis and grossly elevated serum creatine kinase activity. An ECG showed severe hypokalaemic changes, and an electromyogram (EMG) confirmed that she had a myopathy. Muscle biopsy showed moderate atrophy, particularly of the type II fibres. A careful dietary history revealed a low potassium intake and the weekly consumption of up to 1135 g (40 oz) of liquorice sweets. The active ingredient of liquorice is glycyrrhizinic acid which, in large amounts, has a mineralocorticoid effect. It was thought that this, together with a low potassium diet, had led to profound potassium depletion which had been worsened by vomiting and diarrhoea during the preceding influenza-like illness. Once the liquorice was stopped the hypokalaemic alkalosis was corrected by oral and intravenous potassium, the muscle strength improved and the tenderness disappeared.

Myopathic changes

Potassium depletion, however, is not the only reason for muscle weakness. There is now evidence that myopathy and neuropathy may be due to the effects of malnutrition, ipecac poisoning or pressure on peripheral nerves. Essen et al. (1981) carried out muscle biopsies on 10 anorectics who were not complaining of muscle weakness at the time. All muscle fibres showed marked atrophy, but a higher than normal percentage of type 1 fibres was discovered. The percentage of type IIA fibres was normal, but no type IIB fibres were found and, in some patients, there was an increase in the usually rare type IIC fibres. Atrophy of type II fibres has also been reported in other cachectic states (Cullen and Mastaglia, 1982).

Four anorectics who showed no clinical sign of neuromuscular disease were investigated by Lindboe, Askevold and Slettebo (1982). They found atrophy of both type I and type II fibres, but no alteration in the distribution of fibre types. The authors felt that further enquiry was necessary to determine whether the changes they observed were due to malnutrition affecting the muscle fibres directly or the terminations of the nerves supplying them. Accordingly they carried out a further study on 10 new cases of anorexia nervosa and two cachectic females with 'hysterical neurosis' (Slettebo, Lindboe and Askevold, 1984). Five of the anorectics and both the hysterical patients had symptoms and signs of a mild sensory polyneuropathy and had lower body-mass indices (weight divided by the square of the height) than the others. Selective type II atrophy was found in seven of the anorectics and both the hysterics. In addition, the last two cases and two of the anorectics showed muscle biopsy changes consistent with denervation. However, motor nerve conduction velocities were within the normal range. It was concluded that the fibre atrophy was unlikely to be due solely to a neuropathy, but the possibility that it resulted from decreased trophic function of the nerves could not be excluded.

Alloway et al. (1985) have recently described two patients with neuropathy and myopathy. One, a female, suffered from bulimia nervosa; the other was a male with anorexia nervosa. Both complained of weakness. The first found it difficult to climb stairs and had become too weak even to vomit. The second patient was unable to get out of bed. Neither had any symptoms or signs of sensory deficit. On examination there was proximal muscle wasting and weakness, and diminished reflexes. The EMG was abnormal in both patients. A muscle biopsy was carried out in the male anorectic. This again showed atrophy of both type I and type II fibres, the latter predominating.

Ipecac myopathy

Another cause of myopathy in anorexia nervosa is abuse of ipecac to induce vomiting, although to our knowledge this has never been reported in the UK. Brotman et al. (1981) described a patient who consumed up to approximately 300 ml/week of ipecac syrup over a period of 15 months, and large amounts of a laxative for a longer time. While taking ipecac she developed generalized muscle weakness and could barely climb stairs, or even brush her hair. When admitted she was found to have difficulty with both swallowing and speech. Other features were a waddling gait, mild winging of the scapulae, and weakness of the neck flexors and the proximal and distal muscles of all four limbs. The tendon reflexes were sluggish, but coordination was normal and sensation unimpaired. The serum creatine phosphokinase and uric acid levels were elevated, and the EMG showed the appearances of a toxic myopathy with no conduction defect. An asymptomatic but potentially serious finding was an impairment of left ventricular function. After her ipecac and laxatives were stopped, the patient gained weight and all the signs of her myopathy disappeared. Palmer and Guay (1985) have described two further examples, and have pointed out that because of the slow rate of excretion of the active agent, emetine, full recovery and the return of the EMG to normal may take months.

Peripheral nerve compression

Morgan and Russell (1975) and Schott (1979) have reported a further unusual neurological complication of anorexia nervosa, the latter describing a case in detail. A 15-year-old girl presented to a neurological clinic with a 3-month history of difficulty in walking because of right foot drop, and an account of more recent paraesthesia involving the lateral aspect of the lower half of the right leg. She was found to be grossly underweight, but it was only with some difficulty that the diagnosis of anorexia nervosa could be established. The cause of her neurological symptoms turned out to be damage to the common peroneal nerve at the level of the fibular head. In spite of the unilateral nature of her complaints, both legs were affected. It was suggested that loss of protective subcutaneous fat and the patient's inertia were important aetiological factors.

Summary

Neurological manifestations are uncommon with the possible exception of epilepsy, but this does not necessarily imply that there are no underlying abnormalities of the brain and neuromuscular system. Non-specific EEG changes have been found in a high proportion of cases. Reversible cerebral atrophy with dilated lateral ventricles has been demonstrated by computed tomography in a significant number of patients. The relevance of these findings to the disturbed mental state is unclear. Severe muscular weakness is rare and usually associated with potassium depletion, but there is histological evidence of a myopathy in some symptomless patients.

References

ALLOWAY, R., REYNOLDS, E. H., SPARGO, E. and RUSSELL, G. F. M. (1985) Neuropathy and myopathy in two patients with anorexia and bulimia nervosa. *J. Neurol. Neurosurg. Psychiatry*, **48**, 1015–1020

ARTMANN, H., GRAU, H., ADELMAN, M. and SCHLEIFFER, R. (1985) Reversible and non-reversible enlargement of cerebrospinal fluid spaces in anorexia nervosa. *Neuroradiology*, **27**, 304–312

BERANT, M., MANDEL, H. and GOLDSHER, D. (1984) Cerebral and cerebellar atrophy in anorexia nervosa. *Harefuah*, **106**, 212–213

BERGSTROM, K., LUNDBERG, P. O. and SJOVALL, A. (1973) The volume of the sella turcica in patients with anorexia nervosa. *Eur. Neurol.*, **9**, 183–189

BROTMAN, M. C., FORBATH N., GARFINKEL, P. E. and HUMPHREY, J. G. (1981) Myopathy due to ipecac syrup poisoning in a patient with anorexia nervosa. *Can. Med. Assoc. J.*, **125**, 453–454

CALA, L. A. and MASTAGLIA, F. L. (1980) Computerized axial tomography in the detection of brain damage. 1. Alcohol, nutritional deficiency and drugs of addiction. *Med. J. Aust.*, **2**, 193–198

CRISP, A. H., FENTON, G. W. and SCOTTON, L. (1968) A controlled study of the EEG in anorexia nervosa. *Br. J. Psychiatry*, **114**, 1149–1160

CULLEN, M. J. and MASTAGLIA, F. L. (1982) Pathological reactions of skeletal muscle. In *Skeletal Muscle Pathology*, edited by F. L. Mastaglia and J. Walton, pp. 89–139. Edinburgh: Churchill Livingstone

DALLY, P. and SARGANT, W. (1966) Treatment and outcome of anorexia nervosa. *Br. Med. J.*, **2**, 793–795

DATLOF, S., COLEMAN, P. D., FORBES, G. B. and KREIPE, R. E. (1986) Ventricular dilation on CAT scans of patients with anorexia nervosa. *Am. J. Psychiatry*, **143**, 96–98

DUBOIS, F. (1949) Compulsion neurosis with cachexia (anorexia nervosa). *Am. J. Psychiatry*, **106**, 107–115

EMRICH, H. M., PAHL, J. J., HERHOLZ, K., PAWLIK, C., PIRKE, K. M., GERLINGHOFF, M. et al. (1984) PET investigation in anorexia nervosa: normal glucose metabolism during pseudoatrophy of the brain. In *The Psychobiology of Anorexia Nervosa*, edited by K. M. Pirke and D. Ploog, pp. 172–178. Berlin: Springer-Verlag

ENZMANN, D. R. and LANE, B. (1977) Cranial computed tomography findings in anorexia nervosa. *J. Comput. Assist. Tomogr.*, **1**, 410–414

ESSEN, B., FOHLIN, L., THOREN, C. and SALTIN, B. (1981) Skeletal muscle fibre types and sizes in anorexia nervosa patients. *Clin. Physiol.*, **1**, 395–403

FOX, C. F. (1981–82) Neuropsychological correlates of anorexia nervosa. *Int. J. Psychiatry Med.*, **11**, 285–290

GEISLER, E. (1953) Zur Problematik der Pubertatsmagersucht. *Psychiatr. Neurol. Med. Psychol.*, **5**, 227–233

GIBBS, F. A. and GIBBS, E. (1964) *Atlas of Electroencephalography. Vol III*, p. 538. London: Addison-Wesley

GOOR, C. (1954) EEG in anorexia nervosa. *Electroencephalogr. Clin. Neurophysiol.*, **6**, 350

GORDON, D. P., HALMI, K. and IPPOLITO, P. M. (1984) A comparison of the psychological evaluation with anorexia nervosa and of adolescents with conduct disorders. *J. Adolesc.*, **7**, 245–266

GREBB, J. A., YINGLING, C. D. and REUS, V. I. (1984) Electrophysiologic abnormalities in patients with eating disorders. *Compr. Psychiatry*, **25**, 216–224

HALLER, J. O., SLOVIS, T. L., BAKER, D. H., BERDON, W. E. and SILVERMAN, J. A. (1977) Anorexia nervosa—the paucity of radiological findings in more than fifty patients. *Pediatr. Radiol.*, **5**, 145–147

HALMI, K. A. (1974) Anorexia nervosa: demographic and clinical features in 94 cases. *Psychosom. Med.*, **36**, 18–26

HAMSHER, K. DE S., HALMI, K. A. and BENTON, A. L. (1981) Prediction in anorexia nervosa from neurophysiological status. *Psychiatry Res.*, **4**, 79–88

HEIDRICH, R. and SCHMIDT-MATTHIAS, H. (1961) Encephalographische befunde bei Anorexia nervosa. *Archiv fur Psychiatr. Zeitschrift Ges. Neurol.*, **202**, 183–201

HEINZ, E. R., MARTINEZ J. and HAENGGELI, A. (1977) Reversibility of cerebral atrophy in anorexia nervosa and Cushing's syndrome. *J. Comput. Assist. Tomogr.*, **1**, 415–418

KANIS, J. A., BROWN, P., FITZPATRICK, K., HIBBERT, D. J., HORN, D. B., NAIRN, I. M. et al. (1974) Anorexia nervosa: a clinical, psychiatric and laboratory study. *Q. J. Med.*, **67**, 321–328

KOHLMEYER, K., LEHMKUHL, G. and POUTSKA, F. (1983) Computed tomography of anorexia nervosa. *A.J.N.R.*, **4**, 437–438

KRIEG, J.-C., BACKMUND, H. and PIRKE, K.-M. (1987) Cranial computed tomography findings in bulimia. *Acta Psychiatr. Scand.*, **75**, 144–149

LANKENAU, H., SWIGAR, M. E., BHIMANI, S., LUCHINS, D. and QUINLAN, D. M. (1985) Cranial CT scans in eating disorder patients and controls. *Compr. Psychiatry*, **26**, 136–147

LINDBOE, C. F., ASKEVOLD, F. and SLETTEBO, M. (1982) Changes in skeletal muscles of young women with anorexia nervosa. *Acta Neuropathol.*, **56**, 299–302

LUNDBERG, O. and WALINDER, J. (1967) Anorexia nervosa and signs of brain damage. *Int. J. Neuropsychiatr.*, **3**, 165–173

LUTON, J. P., GUILHAUME, B., MARRE, M., FREDY, D. and BRICAIRE, H. (1981) Les anomalies tomodensitometriques cerebrales dans l'anorexie nerveuse. *Nouv. Presse Medicale*, **10**, 1071–1072

MARTIN, F. (1955) Pathologie des aspects neurologiques et psychiatriques dans quelques manifestations carentielles avec troubles digestifs et neuroendocriens. II Etudes des alterations du systeme nerveux central dans deux cas d'anorexie survenue chez la jeune fille (dite anorexie mentale). *Helv. Med. Acta*, **22**, 522–529

MORGAN, H. G. and RUSSELL, G. M. F. (1975) Value of family background and clinical features as predictors of long-term outcome in anorexia nervosa: four-year follow-up study of 41 patients. *Psychol. Med.*, **5**, 355–371

NELL, J. F., MERLKANGAS, J. R., FOSTER, F. G., MERLKANGAS, K. R., SPIKER, D. G. and KUPFER, D. J. (1980) Waking and all-night EEGs in anorexia nervosa. *Clin. Electroencephalogr.*, **11**, 9–15

NIGHTINGALE, S., SMITH, P. E. and TURNBULL, D. M. (1981) Anorexia nervosa, liquorice and hypokalaemic myopathy. *Postgrad. Med. J.*, **57**, 577–579

NUSSBAUM, M., SHENKER, I. R., MARC, J. and KLEIN, M. (1980) Cerebral atrophy in anorexia nervosa. *J. Pediatr.*, **96**, 867–869

PALMER, E. P. and GUAY, A. T. (1985) Reversible myopathy secondary to abuse of ipecac in patients with major eating disorders. *N. Engl. J. Med.*, **313**, 1457–1459

SAUER, H., HORNSTEIN, C. and KESSLER, C. (1985) Irreversible Hirnatrophie bei Anorexia nervosa. *Nervenartz*, **56**, 691–695

SCHOTT, G. D. (1979) Anorexia nervosa presenting as foot drop. *Postgrad. Med. J.*, **55**, 58–60

SEIN, P., SEARSON, S., NICOL, A. R. and HALL, K. (1981) Anorexia nervosa and pseudo-atrophy of the brain. *Br. J. Psychiatry*, **139**, 257–258

SHIMODA, Y. and KITAGAWA, T. (1973) Clinical and EEG studies on the emaciation (anorexia nervosa) due to disturbed function of the brain stem. *J. Neural Transm.*, **34**, 195–204

SILVERMAN, J. A. (1974) Anorexia nervosa: clinical observations in a successful treatment plan. *J. Pediatr.*, **84**, 68–73

SLETTEBO, M., LINDBOE, C. F. and ASKEVOLD, F. (1984) The neuromuscular system in patients with anorexia nervosa: electrophysiological and histologic studies. *Clin. Neurophysiol.*, **3**, 217–224

STRUPP, B. J., WEINGARTNER, H., KAYE, W. and GWIRTSMAN, H. (1986) Cognitive processing in anorexia nervosa. *Neuropsychobiology*, **15**, 89–94

SUEMATSU, H., ISHIWAKA, H., KUBOKI, T. and ITO, T. (1985) Statistical studies on anorexia nervosa in Japan: detailed clinical data on 1011 patients. *Psychother. Psychosom.*, **43**, 96–103

ZEUMER, H., HACKE, W. and HARTWICH, P. (1982) A quantitative approach to measuring the cerebrospinal fluid space with CT. *Neuroradiology*, **22**, 193–197

Chapter 8

The alimentary tract

Gastrointestinal symptoms are not uncommon, but are often difficult to evaluate because they do not always conform to recognized patterns (Berkman, 1930). Nevertheless, abnormalities of the alimentary tract and its associated organs can be demonstrated in some patients. Perusal of the literature suggests that constipation is the commonest complaint. Dysphagia and postprandial nausea or vomiting are also frequently mentioned and meals may be followed by abdominal discomfort. Abdominal pain may however arise unrelated to meals and be ovarian in origin (Crisp, 1985). Some of our patients were found to have polycystic ovaries. Diarrhoea is less common than constipation and should always arouse suspicion of laxative abuse. Vomiting is nearly always self-induced even if this is denied by the patient. Anorectics who have successfully concealed their perverse behaviour from family and close friends usually have little difficulty in doing likewise with inexperienced doctors and nurses. Self-induced vomiting is likely if weight gain fails to occur in spite of an adequate diet, and if frequent visits are made to the toilet, particularly after meals.

Clinical findings

Examination of the abdomen will usually reveal a scaphoid appearance with loss of the subcutaneous fat. Faeces may be palpable through the abdominal wall. Rarely, severe straining may result in haemorrhoids or even rectal prolapse.

The tongue is usually normal, but the teeth may show important changes. Bargen and Austin (1937) described the history and dental findings in a 26-year-old woman with a long history of constipation, reliance on laxatives, and of vomiting after every meal for 6 years. She weighed only 32.7 kg, and was likened to a walking skeleton. Although no diagnosis was given, it is highly likely that the patient had severe anorexia nervosa. Dental examination revealed marked erosion of the teeth and in many places the enamel had completely disappeared. These appearances were attributed to the effects of repeated vomiting. Hellstrom (1977) reported the dental findings in 39 anorectics, of whom 27 were regular vomiters. Dental caries and plaque were present in all, and severe erosion of the lingual–occlusive surface of the teeth was particularly frequent among the vomiters. Hurst, Lacey and Crisp (1977) reviewed the dental condition of 17 anorectics and confirmed the view that vomiting, regurgitation, and eating citrus fruits contribute to loss of enamel. House *et al.* (1981) have advised how the dentist may unmask the surreptitious vomiter and, more recently, Peterson and Barkmeier (1983) published a case of anorexia nervosa where dental pain due to severe erosions was the presenting feature.

Whether or not a patient complains of vomiting, the hands should be closely inspected. Russell (1979) has drawn attention to the presence of raised callosities over the knuckles. These are caused by the teeth as the patient inserts her fingers into the mouth in order to induce vomiting, and in some cases the callosities may actually become ulcerated.

It is not widely recognized that swelling of the salivary glands can occur in this disease, but it must be uncommon for we have seen only one case. The first account was provided by Lavender (1969) who described a 17-year-old male admitted to hospital for investigation of weight loss and bilateral parotid enlargement, his only complaint being dryness of the mouth. He was found to have a hypokalaemic alkalosis, and observed to be vomiting frequently. Further enquiry revealed a history consistent with anorexia nervosa. When last reviewed, the patient had put on weight, his electrolytes were normal and the parotid swelling had virtually disappeared. Dawson and Jones (1977) reported parotid enlargement in a wasted, dehydrated and amenorrhoeic female with a history of vomiting after every meal, and hypokalaemic alkalosis. No cause could be found for the swollen glands, and sialograms showed only diffuse enlargement and normal ducts. As with the first case, the parotids gradually assumed their normal size as the patient's nutritional state improved.

Hasler (1982) described a girl with amenorrhoea who began to diet and developed painful bilateral parotid swelling associated with nausea and vomiting. Extensive investigation failed to reveal any cause for the enlarged glands, and it was well over one year before the patient confessed to regurgitation and self-induced vomiting. In spite of 3 years of treatment she remained thin, and although it appeared that the vomiting had ceased, the parotid glands remained enlarged. The fact that the teeth were in excellent condition may have contributed to the delayed detection of her behaviour.

The patient reported earlier by Bernard and Shearn (1974) was even more devious. On learning that her physicians were considering Sjögren's syndrome as a possible cause of her swollen parotid glands, she looked up the symptoms of this disorder, and successfully fooled a number of doctors into carrying out a plethora of investigations and therapeutic procedures. Her true condition came to light only after a nurse had seen her making herself vomit. The parotids are not the only salivary glands affected in anorexia nervosa; Anders *et al.* (1975) and Kriens *et al.* (1975) have described enlargement of the submandibular and submaxillary glands, respectively.

Special investigations

These are rarely indicated nowadays unless there is doubt over the diagnosis.

Gastric acidity

There was a vogue in the early studies of the pathophysiology of anorexia nervosa for assessing gastric acidity, and it was claimed that achlorhydria was a characteristic of those prone to develop this illness (Surmont, 1920). However, this has not been confirmed (Berkman, 1930; Venables, 1930; McCullagh and Tupper, 1940; Bartels, 1946; Beck and Brochner-Mortensen, 1954).

Radiology

There are a number of published reports of the radiological findings in the alimentary tracts of those suffering from this disease. Ninety-five of the 117 anorectics reported by Berkman (1930) were given barium meals. No abnormality was demonstrated in the majority, but one patient was shown to have a duodenal ulcer, and another had intermittent pyloric obstruction. Beck and Brochner-Mortensen (1954) also found the upper gastrointestinal tract to be normal, apart from one instance of a deformed duodenal cap. In three cases described by Warren and Vande Weile (1973) a barium meal revealed an abnormality. The most serious was in their most wasted patient who began to vomit 2 days after her admission. Investigation revealed a dilated and completely aperistaltic oesophagus. The two other patients had reduced gastric motility, with poor emptying of the stomach, and delayed passage of barium out of the duodenum. Scobie (1972) found that in 10 out of 19 anorectics who had received barium meals the proximal duodenum was shown to be dilated, and there has been a recent report of gastric rugal hypertrophy (Cockett, 1987). Haller et al. (1977) discussed the results of radiological studies carried out on over 50 anorectics in order to exclude other causes of severe weight loss. No oesophageal abnormalities were detected, but in some cases the stomach was enlarged and emptied slowly. One-third of the patients had transient jejunal dilatation, and small bowel transit was occasionally delayed. Ptosis of the transverse colon was a common finding.

Alimentary tract motility

In contrast to a barium meal, manometry may reveal a variety of oesophageal abnormalities. Stacher et al. (1986) investigated 30 patients: seven were found to have achalasia, and eight more had other disturbances of motility. With hindsight it could be argued that the first seven cases did not have anorexia nervosa, since vomiting and loss of weight are not uncommon in achalasia. We have seen a 12-year-old girl with achalasia, misdiagnosed as anorexia nervosa, who gained weight after oesophageal dilatation.

Morlock (1939) regarded delayed gastric emptying as characteristic of anorexia nervosa, and found a fasting gastric content of 200 ml in the case he described; gastroscopy revealed nothing of note, and the secretions were normal in composition. In more recent years, gastric motility has been further studied using special techniques. Silverstone and Russell (1967) measured pressure changes within the stomach to obtain recordings of gastric contractions. Their anorectics, who presented with a variety of feeding patterns, did not differ from healthy controls in terms of either overall gastric motility, or the presence of hunger contractions. Holt et al. (1981), however, demonstrated a reduced rate of gastric emptying in anorectics as compared to healthy subjects, and Dubois, Gross and Ebert (1984) have also shown that gastric emptying is delayed in anorexia nervosa, both under basal conditions and following a water load. Stacher et al. (1986) have demonstrated reduced gastric propulsion of a semi-solid meal.

A more rigorous study is that of McCallum et al. (1985) who pointed out that the proximal stomach or fundus has been shown to regulate the emptying of liquids, whereas the distal stomach, or antrum, controls the emptying of solids. They found that liquid emptying is normal in anorexia nervosa, but solid emptying is slower than in healthy subjects of normal weight. They also confirmed the finding of Saleh and Lebwohl (1980) that metoclopramide accelerated gastric emptying in the anorectics.

The likelihood that intestinal motility is also reduced was raised by Warren and Vande Wiele (1973), who found D-xylose absorption to be reduced in 22% of their patients; there was no evidence of any other cause of malabsorption. Large bowel hypotonia is mentioned below.

Gastrointestinal complications

Various gastrointestinal complications have been described in anorexia nervosa, and may involve the oesophagus, stomach or bowel. The first are rare despite the common practice of self-induced vomiting. The only reported case of oesophageal perforation is that of Schechter, Altemus and Greenfeld (1986), who described a 20-year-old female presenting with severe upper abdominal pain and gross abdominal distension after being unable to make herself sick following binging. Gastric disorders on the other hand are more common.

Gastric dilatation

Russell (1966) provided the earliest description of acute gastric dilatation. The patient, who was known to induce vomiting, had been admitted to hospital and placed on a high-calorie liquid diet which she strongly disliked. She developed what was obviously involuntary vomiting of profuse amounts of greenish fluid; her abdomen became distended, and a succussion splash could be demonstrated. Gastric aspirate produced over 2.5 litres of bile-stained fluid. Water absorption was measured and found to be impaired, suggesting that there was a defect in absorption as well as of motility. As the patient was not hypokalaemic, and others had tolerated the diet well, the author was inclined to attribute the dilatation to psychological factors.

The next case in the literature proved more complicated (Evans, 1968). The patient regained her appetite after receiving chlorpromazine and insulin, but then developed constant abdominal pain and began to vomit. The vomited material became blood-stained, and a laparotomy was carried out. On opening the peritoneum, the stomach, which was grossly distended, ruptured along the anterior surface of the greater curvature. A large infarcted area containing many perforations was discovered. It was suggested that an increase in food intake had resulted in gastric distension, venous occlusion, thrombosis and then infarction.

Two more cases of gastric dilatation were reported by Scobie (1973). Both occurred during refeeding and presented with nausea, abdominal pain and swelling, and absent bowel sounds. The first required a laparotomy and duodenojejunostomy; the second patient, whose stomach contained a bezoar, recovered after conservative management. Subsequent barium studies showed the second patient to have an hour-glass stomach, but gastroscopy showed only an atrophic mucosa. Jennings and Klidjian (1974) presented two further cases, in both of whom gastric dilatation followed an increase in dietary intake. The authors put forward the view that two factors were involved; hypokalaemia in those who regularly vomit, and increased osmolality of the stomach contents following the introduction of relatively large quantities of food and fluid. They did not consider the drugs the patients had been given as a likely cause.

Browning (1977) also emphasized the role of sudden increases in food consumption and described an anorectic who developed gastric dilatation and succumbed to an aspiration pneumonia. At autopsy the stomach was found to have ruptured, but this could have occurred during attempts at resuscitation. His second patient was found at laparotomy to have a gangrenous stomach, and required an oesophagogastrectomy and a jejunostomy. A case where eating almost 1 kg of fruit cake in addition to the normal meal led to gastric dilatation was reported by Brook (1977).

The two anorectics described by Bossingham (1977) are of particular interest in that both deliberately overate in order to be allowed leave over Christmas and Whitsun respectively. The second girl would, on future occasions, overeat in order to provoke the risk of acute gastric dilatation, and hence secure readmission to hospital.

Acute gastric dilatation in the anorectic has been attributed to a variety of causes. These include psychological factors, hypokalaemia and a rapid increase in food intake. The further possibility that duodenal obstruction may be the primary cause is discussed below. Providing the condition is recognized in its early stages, acute gastric dilatation should respond well to nasogastric aspiration and intravenous feeding. If, however, the stomach should rupture, the mortality rate is of the order of 80% (Evans, 1968). Kline (1979) reported that acute dilatation need not be the only cause of rupture, and described a young anorectic girl who had a gastric ulcer which perforated with fatal results.

Intestinal obstruction

Compression of the duodenum by the superior mesenteric artery was described over a century ago, but until relatively recently was thought to occur only rarely in young people. The superior mesenteric artery syndrome, when acute, classically presents with severe postprandial pain and bloating, which is followed by vomiting of bile-stained material. The radiological appearance is of dilatation of the stomach and proximal duodenum. Burrington and Wayne (1974) described 20 patients aged less than 19 years. Three were suffering from anorexia nervosa and presumably had lost the retroperitoneal pad of fat which would normally protect the third part of the duodenum from compression between the superior mesenteric vessels in the root of the mesentery anteriorly, and the aorta and spine posteriorly.

Froese, Szimuilowicz and Bailey (1978) and Sours and Vorhaus (1981) described two further cases arising in anorectics. They stressed that the chronic form may be mistaken for psychogenic vomiting. Pentlow and Dent (1981) presented the case of a 21-year-old anorectic, who denied controlling her weight by vomiting. Eleven days after her admission, by which time she had gained 4 kg, she began to vomit. Over the next 2 days the amount of vomit plus nasogastric aspirate amounted to 5 litres; the diagnosis of postural vascular obstruction to the duodenum was made and a barium meal showed the obstruction to be due to compression by the superior mesenteric artery. The insistence that the girl lay in bed may have been an important contributing factor.

It is surprising that large bowel obstruction seldom occurs, as many patients are severely constipated. We know of only one reported fatality which could have been due to faecal impaction. Kaye, Madden and Leaper (1985) described an emaciated 17-year-old girl who, after being tube-fed for 2 months, developed abdominal colic, constipation, nausea and vomiting. Abdominal radiographs showed a dilated bowel, free peritoneal gas and intraportal venous gas. She was found at laparotomy to have a faecal peritonitis secondary to necrotizing colitis. The patient died shortly afterwards, and at autopsy her rectum was found to be blocked by cement-like faeces.

Other intestinal complications

The effects of chronic laxative abuse on the colon have been discussed by Oster, Materson and Rogers (1980). Melanosis coli, a dark brown-black discoloration of the mucosa and submucosa, is likely to be revealed on endoscopy in those who abuse the anthracene type of laxatives. All evidence points to it being a benign phenomenon which gradually disappears when the purgatives are stopped. A more serious complication is the cathartic colon. The large bowel becomes an inert, dilated, atonic tube incapable of transporting faeces without the aid of large amounts of laxatives. Haustration is lost, and the mucosa becomes smooth and atrophic. Occasionally submucosal retention cysts and superficial punctate ulcerations are present. The stools are usually watery and potassium depletion is a major hazard in these patients.

Liver dysfunction

Cravario, Cravetto and Autino (1974) carried out liver function tests on 27 cases. Serum proteins, transaminases, alkaline phosphatase and bilirubin were normal in every case, as was the response to a bromsulphthalein load. Similarly, Kanis et al. (1974) found that serum aspartate aminotransferase (ASAT) levels were normal in all their 24 anorectics. They also demonstrated, as did Silverman (1974), that protein and albumin levels are not usually reduced in this disease. This is not however a universal finding. For example, Tunbridge and Fraser (1972) described a male anorectic with raised liver enzymes and Steele (1976–77), in his case report of a 19-year-old female who was little over half her ideal weight, stated that she had liver damage, but did not give any details. Nordgren and von Scheele (1977) described an anorectic with biochemical evidence of impaired liver function. There was no history of alcohol abuse, hepatotoxic drugs, or hepatitis to account for this. Her serum ASAT, alanine aminotransferase (ALAT) and lactate dehydrogenase (LDH) concentrations were all raised. A liver biopsy showed non-specific inflammatory infiltrates. The patient was treated with phenothiazines. and electroconvulsive therapy and gained weight slowly. As she did so the serum transaminase and LDH levels fell.

Halmi and Falk (1981) presented the results of liver function tests in 40 anorectics investigated before, during and after treatment. Some of their patients had raised concentrations of serum ASAT, LDH and alkaline phosphatase, but the serum bilirubin concentrations, protein levels and prothrombin times were normal. Garfinkel and Garner (1982) reported that 6% of their cases had elevated serum ASAT concentrations. More striking abnormalities were reported by Milner, McAnarney and Klish (1985) in a group of underweight children and adolescents, but we are not convinced that all their patients were suffering from anorexia nervosa. For example, the youngest was only 7 years old.

Various liver function tests were carried out on 83 of our drug-free patients. Serum albumin levels were measured in 82 and were found to be elevated in 21 (26%). Serum ASAT concentrations were raised in 29 out of 79 cases (37%). One of these had a level of 1095 IU/l. There was no obvious explanation for this gross increase and the level fell to normal as she put on weight. The serum ALAT level was measured in only 20 drug-free patients, but was found to be increased in four, the highest value being 91 IU/l. Increases in the serum bilirubin, alkaline phosphatase and γ-glutamyltransferase levels were less frequently encountered and were usually moderate.

Pancreatic disorders

As long ago as 1936 Ryle reported that one of his fatal cases was found to have an atrophied pancreas. More recently Nordgren and von Scheele (1977) described a young woman with a 5-year history of anorexia nervosa, and a 2-year history of abdominal pain. Both serum and urinary amylase levels were raised, but cholecystography, radioisotope pancreatic scan, duodenoscopy and pancreatic ductography revealed nothing abnormal. As she gained weight the amylase concentrations fell to normal. The patient later relapsed and, as she lost weight, the serum amylase level rose once again. Cox et al. (1983) recently investigated 10 unselected cases and found that seven had raised amylase/creatinine clearance ratios. Three had elevated serum amylase levels and three were discovered to have diminished pancreatic density on ultrasound examination. However, none of the patients showed any clinical evidence of pancreatic disease or dysfunction.

Acute pancreatitis may occasionally occur during the course of treatment. Keane, Fennell and Tomkin (1978) described the association of acute pancreatitis, acute gastric dilatation, and duodenal ileus in a single case. They suggested that the primary abnormality could have been duodenal compression by the superior mesenteric artery which in turn led to duodenal ileus and reflux into the pancreatic ducts. Gryboski et al. (1980) reported two anorectics who as the result of coming into hospital, doubled their daily calorie intake. The first, a 17-year-old boy, experienced constant epigastric pain 24 hours after admission. His condition rapidly deteriorated and abdominal examination revealed an enlarged liver, marked epigastric tenderness and diminished bowel sounds. The serum amylase, lipase and liver enzyme levels were raised. The second patient was a 14-year-old girl who developed symptoms on her third day of refeeding. As with the first case, she became acutely ill and had clinical and biochemical signs of acute pancreatitis. The radiological findings were consistent with compression of the duodenum by the superior mesenteric artery. A similar mechanism may have accounted for the concurrence of pancreatitis and acute gastric dilatation in the patient reported by Backett (1985), as both the stomach and duodenal cap were markedly distended.

Summary

Anorexia nervosa affects the alimentary tract in a number of ways. The more benign manifestations such as dental caries and enlarged salivary glands may lead to the discovery of surreptitious vomiting. The evaluation of the more serious complications calls for considerable clinical acumen as most present with vomiting and abdominal pain. There is the risk, particularly with the uncooperative patient, that the vomiting will be assumed mistakenly to be self-induced, and that complaints of nausea or abdominal pain will be seen as just another attempt to avoid eating. Constipation is so common that laxative abuse should always be suspected if the stools are loose. The cause of the disturbed liver function tests in some patients is unknown, but they usually revert to normal on refeeding. Pancreatic disorders appear to be less frequent, and some may be due to compression of the duodenum by the superior mesenteric artery.

References

ANDERS, D., HARMS, D., KRIENS, O. and SCHMIDT, H. (1975) Zur frage der sialadenose als sekundarer organmanifestation der anorexia nervosa—beobachtungen an einem 13-jahrigen knaben. *Klin. Padiatr.*, **187**, 156–162

BACKETT, S. A. (1985) Acute pancreatitis and gastric dilatation in a patient with anorexia nervosa. *Postgrad. Med. J.*, **61**, 39–40

BARGEN, J. A. and AUSTIN, L. T. (1937) Decalcification of teeth as a result of obstipation with long continued vomiting: report of a case. *J. Am. Dent. Assoc.*, **24**, 1271–1273

BARTELS, E. D. (1946) Studies on hypometabolism I: anorexia nervosa. *Acta Med. Scand.*, **124**, 185–211

BECK, J. C. and BROCHNER-MORTENSEN, K. (1954) Observations on the prognosis in anorexia nervosa. *Acta Med. Scand.*, **149**, 409–430

BERKMAN, J. M. (1930) Anorexia nervosa, anorexia, inanation, and low basal metabolic rate. *Am. J. Med. Sci.*, **180**, 411–424

BERNARD, J. D. and SHEARN, M. A. (1974) Psychogenic pseudo-Sjögren's syndrome. *West J. Med.*, **120**, 247–248

BOSSINGHAM, D. (1977) Acute gastric dilatation in anorexia nervosa. *Br. Med. J.*, ii, 959

BROOK, G. K. (1977) Acute gastric dilatation in anorexia nervosa. *Br. Med. J.*, ii, 499–500

BROWNING, C. H. (1977) Anorexia nervosa: complications of somatic therapy. *Compr. Psychiatry*, **18**, 399–403

BURRINGTON, J. D. and WAYNE, F. R. (1974) Obstruction of the duodenum by the superior mesenteric artery—does it exist in children? *J. Pediatr. Surg.*, **9**, 733–741

COCKETT, A. D. (1987) Anorexia nervosa and gastric rugal hyperplasia. *Br. J. Psychiatry*, **150**, 697–700

COX, K. L., CANNON, R. A., AMENT, M. E., PHILLIPS, H. E. and SCHAFFER, C. B. (1983) Biochemical and ultrasonic abnormalities of the pancreas in anorexia nervosa. *Dig. Dis. Sci.*, **28**, 225–229

CRAVARIO, A., CRAVETTO, C. A. and AUTINO, R. (1974) Studio della funzionalita epatica nell' anoressia nervosa. *Minerva Med.*, **65**, 2990–2995

CRISP, A. H. (1985) Gastrointestinal disturbance in anorexia nervosa. *Postgrad. Med. J.*, **61**, 3–5

DAWSON, J. and JONES, C. (1977) Vomiting-induced hypokalaemic alkalosis and parotid swelling. *Practitioner*, **218**, 267–268

DUBOIS, A., GROSS, H. A. and EBERT, M. H. (1984) Gastric function in primary anorexia nervosa. In: *The Psychobiology of Anorexia Nervosa*, edited by D. M. Pirke and D. Ploog, pp. 87–92. Berlin: Springer-Verlag

EVANS, D. S. (1968) Acute dilatation and spontaneous rupture of the stomach. *Br. J. Surg.*, **55**, 940–942

FROESE, A. P., SZIMUILOWICZ, J. and BAILEY, J. D. (1978) The superior-mesenteric-artery syndrome: cause or complication of anorexia nervosa. *Can. Psychiatr. Assoc J.*, **23**, 325–327

GARFINKEL, R. M. and GARNER, P. E. (1982) *Anorexia Nervosa: a Multidimensional Perspective*, p. 320. New York: Brunner/Mazel.

GRYBOSKI, J., HILLMEIER, C., KOCOSHIS, S., ANYAN, W. and SEASHORE, J. S. (1980) Refeeding pancreatitis in malnourished children. *J. Pediatr.*, **97**, 441–443

HALLER, J. O., SLOVIS, T. L., BAKER, D. H., BERDON, W. E. and SILVERMAN, J. A. (1977) Anorexia nervosa—the paucity of radiological findings in more than fifty patients. *Pediatr. Radiol.*, **5**, 145–147

HALMI, K. A. and FALK, J. R. (1981) Common physiological changes in anorexia nervosa. *Int. J. Eating Disorders*, **1**, 16–27

HASLER, J. F. (1982) Parotid enlargement: a presenting sign in anorexia nervosa. *Oral Surg.*, **53**, 567–573

HELLSTROM, I. (1977) Oral complications in anorexia nervosa. *Scand. J. Dent. Res.*, **85**, 71–86

HOLT, S., FORD, M. J., GRANT, S. and HEADING, R. C. (1981) Abnormal gastric emptying in primary anorexia nervosa. *Br. J. Psychiatry*, **139**, 550–552

HOUSE, R. C., GRISIUS, R., BLIZIOTES, M. M. and LICHT, J. H. (1981) Perimolysis: unveiling the surreptitious vomiter. *Oral Surg.*, **51**, 152–155

HURST, P. S., LACEY, J. H. and CRISP, A. H. (1977) Teeth, vomiting and diet: a study of the dental characteristics of seventeen anorexia nervosa patients. *Postgrad. Med. J.*, **53**, 298–305

JENNINGS, K. P. and KLIDJIAN, A. M. (1974) Acute gastric dilatation in anorexia nervosa. *Br. Med. J.*, ii, 477–478

KANIS, J. A., BROWN, P., FITZPATRICK, K., HIBBERT, D. J., HORN, D. B., NAIRN, I. M. et al. (1974) Anorexia nervosa: a clinical, psychiatric and laboratory study. *Q. J. Med.*, **67**, 321–328

KAYE, J. C., MADDEN, M. V. and LEAPER, D. J. (1985) Anorexia nervosa and necrotizing colitis. *Postgrad. Med. J.*, **61**, 41–42

KEANE, F. B. V., FENNELL, J. S. and TOMKIN, G. H. (1978) Acute pancreatitis, acute gastric dilatation and duodenal ileus following refeeding in anorexia nervosa. *Ir. J. Med. Sci.*, **147**, 191–192

KLINE, C. L. (1979) Anorexia nervosa: death from complications of ruptured gastric ulcer. *Can. J. Psychiatry*, **24**, 153–156

KRIENS, O., SCHMIDT, H., ANDERS, D. and HARMS, D. (1975) Sialadenose bei einem jungen mit anorexia nervosa. *Dtsch. Zahnaertzl Z.*, **30**, 547–551

LAVENDER, S. (1969) Vomiting and parotid enlargement. *Lancet*, i, 426

MCCALLUM, R. W., GRILL, B. B., LANGE, R., PLANKY, M., GLASS, E. and GREENFELD, D. G. (1985) Definition of a gastric emptying abnormality in patients with anorexia nervosa. *Dig. Dis. Sci.*, **30**, 713–722

MCCULLAGH, E. P. and TUPPER, W. R. (1940) Anorexia nervosa. *Ann. Int. Med.*, **14**, 817–838

MILNER, M. R., MCANARNEY, E. R. and KLISH, W. J. (1985) Metabolic abnormalities in adolescent patients with anorexia nervosa. *J. Adolesc. Health Care.*, **6**, 193–195

MORLOCK, C. G. (1939) Anorexia nervosa. *Proc. Staff Meet. Mayo Clin.*, **14**, 24–28

NORDGREN, I. and VON SCHEELE, C. (1977) Hepatic and pancreatic dysfunction in anorexia nervosa: a report of two cases. *Biol. Psychiatry*, **12**, 681–686

OSTER, J. R., MATERSON, B. J. and ROGERS, A. I. (1980) Laxative abuse syndrome. *Am. J. Gastroenterol.*, **74**, 451–458

PENTLOW, B. D. and DENT, R. G. (1981) Acute vascular compression of the duodenum in anorexia nervosa. *Br. J. Surg.*, **68**, 665–666

PETERSON, D. S. and BARKMEIER, W. W. (1983) Oral signs of frequent vomiting in anorexia. *Am. Fam. Physician*, **27**, 199–200

RUSSELL, G. (1979) Bulimia nervosa: an ominous variant of anorexia nervosa. *Psychol. Med.*, **4**, 429–448

RUSSELL, G. F. M. (1966) Acute dilatation of the stomach in a patient with anorexia nervosa. *Br. J. Psychiatry*, **112**, 203–207

RYLE, J. A. (1936) Anorexia nervosa. *Lancet*, ii, 893–899

SALEH, J. W. and LEBWOHL, P. (1980) Metoclopramide-induced gastric emptying in patients with anorexia nervosa. *Am. J. Gastroenterol.*, **74**, 127–132

SCHECHTER, J. O., ALTEMUS, M. and GREENFELD, D. G. (1986) Food bingeing and esophageal perforation in anorexia nervosa. *Hosp. Community Psychiatry*, **37**, 507–508

SCOBIE, B. A. (1972) Acute dilatation of the stomach in patients with anorexia nervosa. *Aust. N.Z. J. Med.*, **3**, 335

SCOBIE, B. A. (1972) Acute gastric dilatation and duodenal ileus in anorexia nervosa. *Med. J. Aust.*, **2**, 932–934

SILVERMAN, J. A. (1974) Anorexia nervosa: clinical observations in a successful treatment plan. *J. Pediatr.*, **84**, 68–73

SILVERSTONE, J. T. and RUSSELL, G. F. M. (1967) Gastric 'hunger' contractions in anorexia nervosa. *Br. J. Psychiatry*, **13**, 257–263

SOURS, J. A. and VORHAUS, L. J. (1981) Superior mesenteric artery syndrome in anorexia nervosa: a case report. *Am. J. Psychiatry*, **138**, 519–520

STACHER, G., KISS, A., WIESNAGROTZKI, S., BERGMAN, H., HOBART, J. and SCHNEIDER, C. (1986) Oesophageal and gastric motility disorders in patients categorised as having primary anorexia nervosa. *Gut*, **27**, 1120–1126

STEELE, R. L. (1976–77) Anorexia nervosa: a case study. *Psychother. Psychosom.*, **27**, 47–53

SURMONT, H. (1920) Les diverse formes de l'anorexie nerveuse: leur diagnostic. *Medecine*, **1**, 603–605

TUNBRIDGE, W. M. G. and FRASER, T. R. (1972) Anorexia nervosa with multiple disorders in a young man. *Proc. R. Soc. Med.*, **65**, 21–21

VENABLES, J. F. (1930) Anorexia nervosa: a study of the pathogenesis and treatment of nine cases. *Guy's Hospital Reports*, **80**, 213–226

WARREN, M. P. and VANDE WIELE, R. L. (1973) Clinical and metabolic features of anorexia nervosa. *Am. J. Obstet. Gynecol.*, **117**, 435–449

Chapter 9

Haematology and immunology

It is often stated that the blood picture is normal in anorexia nervosa. For example, Kanis *et al.* (1974) found in their series that both haemoglobin levels and leucocyte counts were as expected in a healthy population. Our experience and that of others suggests that this is not always so. Among the many changes that have been described are anaemia, leucopenia, lymphopenia, thrombocytopenia, decreased granulocyte bactericidal activity, and decreased polymorphonuclear leucocyte adherence. In addition, hypocomplementaemia and increased plasminogen activator activity have been described, as well as alterations in cell-mediated immunological mechanisms.

Peripheral blood

The first systematic study of the peripheral blood in anorexia nervosa was probably that of Carryer, Berkman and Mason (1959) who reviewed 26 cases. Haemoglobin levels ranged from 1.6 to 2.7 mmol/l (10.4–17.2 g/dl), but nine patients had white cell counts of less than 5.0×10^9/l. Of these, four had counts of 4.0×10^9/l or less, the lowest value being 2.7×10^9/l. There was a relative lymphocytosis due to a reduction in the polymorphonuclear count. No comment was made regarding the platelets. The authors noted that their findings were consistent with earlier reports on the affects of involuntary starvation.

Haemoglobin levels

Anaemia is uncommon in anorexia nervosa and is usually mild. Warren and Vande Wiele (1973) reported that only three of their 42 cases were anaemic, the red cells being normochromic and normocytic. Lampert and Lau (1976) found no anaemia among their anorectics and noted high haemoglobin levels, possibly due to dehydration, in half of them. By contrast, Mant and Faragher (1972) reported that five of their six cases were anaemic when at their lowest weights. Haemoglobin levels were measured in 97 of our patients before they were put on any medication. They ranged from 1.6 to 2.6 mmol/l (10.2–16.7 g/dl), but were lower than 1.9 mmol/l (12.0 g/dl) in only nine cases. A transient fall in the haematocrit and haemoglobin level is not uncommon at the onset of treatment, and possibly reflects rehydration (Mant and Faragher, 1972; Bowers and Eckert, 1978; Halmi and Falk, 1981).

The mean corpuscular haemoglobin concentration, the mean corpuscular haemoglobin content and the mean red cell volume are usually all normal (Halmi and Falk,

1981), but Mant and Faragher (1972) reported the presence of anisocytes, poikilocytes and particularly acanthocytes. The large number of acanthocytes in this disease was confirmed by Cornbleet, Moir and Wolf (1977) who pointed out that similar red cells are seen in hereditary abetalipoproteinaemia. This fitted in with the suggestion of Mant and Faragher that low levels of beta-lipoprotein may be responsible. Amrein *et al.* (1979) described an anaemic anorectic who succumbed to an infection. Nearly all her red cells were acanthocytes and no beta-lipoprotein could be found on protein electrophoresis. Two possible explanations of acanthocytosis were mentioned. One was that the low beta-lipoprotein concentration results in inefficient removal of cholesterol from the cells, leading to redundant cell membrane and hence spiculation. The alternative view was that red blood cell viscosity is lost due to a high cholesterol/phospholipid ratio in low-density lipoproteins.

Mant and Faragher (1972) and Casper *et al.* (1980) found serum iron levels to be normal in their cases, but iron binding capacity was reduced. There is, however, one report of iron deficiency being so marked as to cause not only severe anaemia, but also the Paterson–Brown–Kelly syndrome (Evans, 1939).

White cell counts

That leucopenia may occur in anorexia nervosa has been confirmed on a number of occasions. Even when within the normal range the white cell count tends to be lower than in healthy persons of comparable race, sex, age and social class (Reiger, Brady and Weisberg, 1978). Mant and Faragher (1972) found that half their cases had white cell counts of below $5.0 \times 10^9/l$. The corresponding figure in the 42 patients of Warren

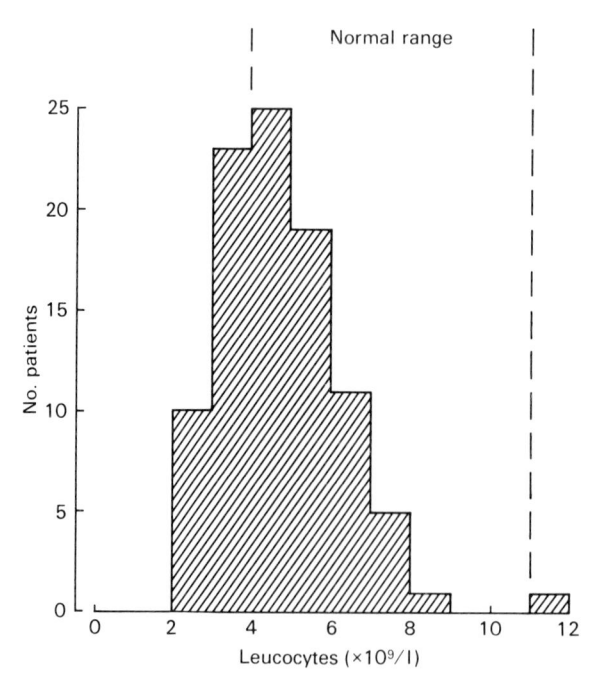

Figure 9.1 Distribution of total white cell counts in 95 untreated patients; 31% had counts below $4.0 \times 10^9/l$

and Vande Wiele (1973) was 38%, the lowest white cell count being $2.0 \times 10^9/l$. One patient had been previously thought to have glandular fever or a viral hepatitis, and another a leukaemia. Six patients had a relative lymphocytosis. Silverman (1974) reported the incidence of leucopenia as 24%, and in the smaller series of Lampert and Lau (1976) and Smith and Spivak (1985) it was 60% and 66% respectively. Thirty-one per cent of our 95 drug-free patients had white cell counts below $4.0 \times 10^9/l$ (*Figure 9.1*).

Halmi and Falk (1981) presented their data in summary form only, but observed that, with successful treatment, the white cell count increases and the relative lymphocytosis disappears. However, leucopenia in anorexia nervosa may be iatrogenic. Pisciotta (1969) pointed out that phenothiazine-induced agranulocytosis may occur at any time between 10 and 70 days, and is often asymptomatic in the early stages. He recommended weekly leucocyte counts as a routine. If the white count should fall, and the cause be in doubt, marrow studies should clarify the situation.

Platelet counts

Thrombocytopenia can occur in anorexia nervosa, but is usually described as being rare. Although Mant and Faragher (1972) and Lampert and Lau (1976) reported a relatively high incidence, most authors mention only single instances (Warren and Vande Wiele, 1973; Silverman, 1974; Amrein *et al.*, 1979; Brotman and Stern, 1983; Marechaud *et al.*, 1985; Smith and Spivak, 1985). Most of these cases had purpura, ecchymoses or both; in addition, the severely ill patient of Amrein *et al.* (1979) had blood oozing from her nose. In our series platelet counts were not requested as a matter of routine, but in the more recent cases were made available through automated blood analysis. In the 37 anorectics who were not on medication the platelet count ranged from 77 to $423 \times 10^9/l$. Only three were thrombocytopenic, their platelet counts being 77, 104 and $141 \times 10^9/l$ respectively.

Bone marrow

The bone marrow was first investigated in anorexia nervosa by Pearson (1967) who reported on three cases. None were anaemic, although in one patient ferrokinetic studies indicated reduced erythropoiesis, and two had normal white cell counts. The third case had a persistent leucopenia in spite of a chest infection. The marrows were all hypoplastic, with a marked dearth of haematopoietic cells and an increase in acid mucopolysaccharide ground substance. These findings were confirmed by Mant and Faragher (1972) in five patients. It was noted that, in addition to hypocellularity and increased ground substance, there was a loss of marrow fat and histiocytes containing blue-green granules were present. There was no evidence of iron, vitamin B_{12}, or folate deficiency. A further seven anorectics were investigated by Lampert and Lau (1976), with similar findings. In five cases haemoglobin levels and haematocrits were normal, in spite of a noticeable lack of erythroblasts.

Tavassoli *et al.* (1976) reported the findings in three cases of prolonged self-starvation, two of whom were strict vegetarians. The youngest was 52 years old and none of the histories were typical of anorexia nervosa. One was anaemic, two had leucopenia, and all three had low serum albumin levels. Nevertheless, the marrow findings resembled those seen in anorectics. Similar abnormalities were produced in laboratory rabbits on restricted diets for 4 months; as with anorectics, refeeding resulted in the marrow recovering. Cornbleet, Moir and Wolf (1977) and Smith and Spivak (1985) have compared the marrow appearances in anorectics with those in patients with organic cachexia, and have found them to be similar.

Smith and Spivak (1985) were also the first to report marrow cell necrosis in anorexia nervosa. This was limited to the areas where the mucopolysaccharide was present. They suggested that gelatinous transformation and cell necrosis represent opposite reactions to the rate of bone marrow starvation. When this occurs gradually, as in anorexia nervosa, the former is seen; however, if the supply of nutrients is abruptly interfered with, as might happen in infections, cell necrosis results.

The extent and clinical significance of marrow hypoplasia in anorexia nervosa can be judged from the reports of Warren and Vande Wiele (1973) and Silverman (1974). The first found that six out of 13 anorectics had hypoplastic marrows, but only two of them had any peripheral haematological abnormality. Silverman (1974) noted abnormal marrows in 41% of his cases, and leucopenia in only 24%. However, life-threatening pancytopenia may occur (Amrein *et al.*, 1979; Marechaud *et al.*, 1985), and particular vigilance is called for if the patients should develop an infection or adverse drug reaction. A marrow biopsy was abnormal in all five of our patients in whom this procedure was carried out, the findings being similar to those described. One case almost succumbed to an overwhelming infection with only a minimal rise in her white cell count.

The erythrocyte sedimentation rate

The erythrocyte sedimentation rate (ESR) is frequently used as a screening test for organic pathology. Anyan (1974) measured the ESR and plasma fibrinogen level in 22 young females and five boys who had anorexia nervosa. The ESRs tended to be toward the lower end of the normal range, as did the fibrinogen levels. After recovery, the ESRs and fibrinogen levels rose. The author attributed the reduced ESR in anorexia nervosa to the presence of acanthocytes, which sediment slowly, and the relatively low plasma fibrinogen levels. That the ESR response to illness can still take place was shown by one of the patients who developed pneumonia; there was no fever or leucocytosis but the ESR increased to 51 mm/h. The ESR was initially normal in all our cases, but showed a modest rise in those with intercurrent infection.

Ogston and Ogston (1976) confirmed the presence of low fibrinogen levels in anorectics, and also reported that plasminogen activator levels were increased. The mean levels of plasminogen, fibrin degradation products, and the major antiplasmins did not differ from those in the healthy controls. Whatever the cause and significance of these findings, it appears that they have usually no effect on bleeding time or clot retraction (Halmi and Falk, 1981).

Responses to infection

Pearson (1967) regarded the haematological abnormalities occurring in anorexia nervosa as laying the patient open to an increased risk of infection. Bowers and Eckert (1978) compared 68 anorectics with 68 psychiatric patients matched for sex and age, and found that the anorectics had lower total white cell, neutrophil, lymphocyte and monocyte counts. However, the neutrophil response to hydrocortisone suggested that the neutrophil reserves in the patients were normal. Twelve instances of infection were recorded among the control group, but only seven among the anorectics. The authors concluded that, if there is an increased risk of infection among anorectics, it is not due solely to leucopenia, and other explanations must be considered.

Gotch et al. (1975) described three anorectics who had leucopenia. Their granulocytes were found to have reduced bactericidal activity when incubated with *Staphylococcus aureus* and *Escherichia coli*. IgG opsonization of *S. aureus* was normal and there appeared to be no defect in phagocytosis. One patient suffered from recurrent abdominal abscesses. After she gained weight her granulocyte function returned to normal and her infection cleared despite the fact that she was still neutropenic. Palmblad, Fohlin and Lundstrom (1977) also demonstrated impaired granulocyte bactericidal capacity, and noted reduced granulocyte adherence. The mean chemotaxis did not differ between the anorectics and the controls, but in two anorectics chemotaxis was virtually absent. None of their 10 patients, however, suffered from severe or recurrent infections.

The complement system

Silverman (1974) reported that immunoglobulin levels were normal in anorectics. By contrast, Kim and Micheal (1975) described hypocomplementaemia in a male anorectic prone to recurrent staphylococcal skin infections. There was a significant reduction in the serum concentrations of C1, C2, C3, C1s inactivator, factor B and total haemolytic complement. By the time he had regained weight the serum levels of all complement components were normal and presumably the skin infections had stopped. Similar findings of deficiencies in complement (C1q, C2–C6, factor B and properdin) and their control proteins (β-1H, C3b1NA and C4bp) were described in five anorectics without infection (Wyatt et al., 1982). The frequency of complement deficiencies remains to be determined, as Murphy et al. (1985) from the same group described a single severe case in which levels of complement components were normal.

The presence of infections in patients makes it difficult to determine which of three alternative defects results in low complement levels: a low rate of protein synthesis, inactivation of complement enzyme function, or rapid removal from the circulation. Wyatt et al. (1982) argued convincingly that in anorectics without infections low serum levels of the complement regulatory proteins β-1H and C3b1NA are due to a low synthetic rate. As a consequence of prior synthesis of regulatory proteins, C3 and factor B levels are low because of an increased turnover of the C3b amplification loop. In Wyatt's patients, all four complement components rose rapidly with refeeding. Although it is accepted that an intact complement system is important for host defence against infection, the difference between anorectics, who in general are not prone to infections, and malnourished children who are, may be the consequence of increased exposure to pathogenic organisms rather than low rates of synthesis of complement components.

Armstrong-Esther et al. (1978) commented on the fact that anorectics rarely contract the common cold or influenza and compared the responses of anorectics and an age and occupation-matched control group to vaccination against influenza. At first both had similar haemagglutination inhibition titres against the three antigens (A/HK, A/PC, and A/Eng), but during the next 2 months the anorectics showed higher titres, particularly to the Hong Kong virus. By contrast, George (1981) reported herpes simplex encephalitis, a condition often associated with impaired immune mechanisms, occurring in a case of anorexia nervosa.

Cell-mediated immunity

There appears to be some impairment of cell-mediated immunity in many anorectics but it is difficult to determine from the rather scanty literature which components are defective. Delayed hypersensitivity reactions *in vivo* (anergy) have been measured in several studies but with differing results. For example Armstrong-Esther *et al.* (1978) reported little difference in the incidence of positive tuberculin tests between anorectics (53%) and controls (67%). However, the amount of carbohydrates ingested by the fifteen patients at the time of testing varied considerably. Two other studies of anergy were uncontrolled. In one of these, four out of eight cases were virtually anergic (Golla *et al.*, 1981). In the other study six out of 22 patients were anergic and anergy was significantly related to indicators of malnutrition such as weight loss (Pertschuk *et al.*, 1982). In a more recent and better designed study, delayed hypersensitivity reactions to 1% *Candida albicans*, 10 u purified protein derivative, 3% tricophytin and varidase were noticeably less evident in the anorectics as compared with healthy control subjects. Reduction in erythema was more striking than reduction in induration (Cason *et al.*, 1986).

Although other methods of measuring cell-mediated immunity suggest that components are low or functions reduced in some cases, none of these measurements demonstrate statistically significant impairment. Indeed, Golla *et al.* (1981) found normal T-lymphocyte populations and a significantly greater proliferative response to mitogenic stimuli in nine anorectics compared with controls, although the lymphocyte proliferative response decreased when weight was regained. However, only a single dose of each mitogen was tested. Cason *et al.* (1986) suggested that this dose would have been supra-optimal if a dose-response curve had been established. These authors also compared anorectics and controls for lymphocyte transformation and found higher doses were required to elicit a comparable response among the anorectics. They also found that mononuclear cells and polymorph counts were similar in patients and controls, and the lower numbers of T3 and T4 positive cells in the anorectics and the increase in T8 positive cells in the controls failed to reach statistical significance. Despite this, they concluded that there are functional cellular abnormalities associated with undernutrition in this condition. Finally, Wade *et al.* (1985) have found significantly reduced activity of the thymic hormone, thymulin, in anorectics and suggest that this could account for their variability in cellular immune responses.

Summary

In spite of the various haematological and immunological changes in anorexia nervosa, it appears that anorectics are less vulnerable to infection than are those suffering from other forms of malnutrition and weight loss. However, should an anorectic acquire an infection the results may be serious. It could be argued from this that the early stages of defence by the immune system function normally to prevent infection in most anorectic patients. Examples of these early stages are phagocytosis and complement-mediated opsonization. However, if an infection overcomes the patient's initial barriers, later-acting defence mechanisms, such as intracellular killing by granulocytes and cell-mediated immunity, may be impaired and permit the infection to become firmly established.

References

AMREIN, P. C., FRIEDMAN, R., KOSINSKI, K. and ELLMAN, L. (1979) Hematologic changes in anorexia nervosa. *J. Am. Med. Assoc.*, **241**, 2190–2191

ANYAN, W. R. (1974) Changes in erythrocyte sedimentation rate and fibrinogen during anorexia nervosa. *J. Pediatr.*, **85**, 525–527

ARMSTRONG-ESTHER, C. A., LACEY, J. H., CRISP, A. H. and BRYANT, T. N. (1978) An investigation of the immune response of patients suffering from anorexia nervosa. *Postgrad. Med. J.*, **54**, 395–399

BOWERS, T. K. and ECKERT, E. (1978) Leukopenia in anorexia nervosa. *Arch. Intern. Med.*, **138**, 1520–1523

BROTMAN, A. W. and STERN, T. A. (1983) Case report of cardiovascular abnormalities in anorexia nervosa. *Am. J. Psychiatry*, **140**, 1227–1228

CARRYER, H. M., BERKMAN, J. M. and MASON, H. L. (1959) Relative lymphocytosis in anorexia nervosa. *Proc. Staff Meetings Mayo Clin.*, **34**, 426–432

CASON, J., AINLEY, C. C., WOLSTENCROFT, R. A., NORTON, K. R. W. and THOMPSON, R. P. H. (1986) Cell-mediated immunity in anorexia nervosa. *Clin. Exp. Immunol.*, **64**, 370–375

CASPER, R. C., KIRSCHNER, B., SANDSTEAD, H. H., JACOB, R. A. and DAVIS, J. M. (1980) An evaluation of trace metals, vitamins, and taste function in anorexia nervosa. *Am. J. Clin. Nutr.*, **33**, 1801–1808

CORNBLEET, P. J., MOIR, R. C. and WOLF, P. L. (1977) A histochemical study of bone marrow hypoplasia in anorexia nervosa. *Virchows Arch.* (A), **374**, 239–247

EVANS, J. C. G. (1939) Anorexia nervosa. *Lancet*, i, 268–269

GEORGE, G. K. W. (1981) Anorexia nervosa with herpes simplex encephalitis. *Postgrad. Med. J.*, **57**, 366–367

GOLLA, J. A., LARSON, L. A., ANDERSON, C. F., LUCAS, A. R., WILSON, W. R. and TOMASI, T. B. (1981) An immunological assessment of patients with anorexia nervosa. *Am. J. Clin. Nutr.*, **34**, 2756–2762

GOTCH, F. M., SPRY, C. J. F., MOWAT, A. G., BEESON, P. B. and MACLENNAN, I. C. M. (1975) Reversible granulocyte killing defect in anorexia nervosa. *Clin. Exp. Immunol.*, **21**, 244–249

HALMI, K. A. and FALK, J. R. (1981) Common physiological changes in anorexia nervosa. *Int. J. Eating Disorders*, **1**, 16–27

KANIS, J. A., BROWN, P., FITZPATRICK, K., HIBBERT, D. J., HORN, D. B., NAIRN, I. M. et al. (1974) Anorexia nervosa: a clinical, psychiatric and laboratory study. *Q. J. Med.*, **67**, 321–328

KIM, Y. and MICHEAL, A. F. (1975) Hypocomplementemia in anorexia nervosa. *J. Pediatr.*, **87**, 582–585

LAMPERT, F. and LAU, B. (1976) Bone marrow hypoplasia in anorexia nervosa. *Eur. J. Pediatr.*, **124**, 65–71

MANT, M. J. and FARAGHER, B. S. (1972) The haematology of anorexia nervosa. *Br. J. Haematol.*, **23**, 737–749

MARECHAUD, R., ABADIE, J. C., BABIN, P., LESSART, M. and SUDRE, Y. (1985) Hypoplasie medullaire reversible au cours d'une anorexie mentale masculine. *Ann. Med. Interne*, **136**, 36–40

MURPHY, D. J., DICKSON, T. M., BRUNNER, R. L., MALONEY, M. J., FARRELL M. K., MEYER, R. A. et al. (1985) Concomitant psychological improvement during successful treatment of anorexia nervosa. *J. Adolesc. Health Care*, **6**, 392–396

OGSTON, D. and OGSTON, W. D. (1976) The fibrinolytic enzyme system in anorexia nervosa. *Acta Haematol.*, **55**, 230–233

PALMBLAD, J., FOHLIN, L. and LUNDSTROM, M. (1977) Anorexia nervosa and polymorphonuclear (PMN) granulocyte reactions. *Scand. J. Haematol.*, **19**, 334–342

PEARSON, H. A. (1967) Marrow hypoplasia in anorexia nervosa. *J. Pediatr.*, **71**, 211–215

PERTSCHUK, M. J., CROSBY, L. O., BAROT, L. and MULLEN, J. L. (1982) Immunocompetency in anorexia nervosa. *Am. J. Clin. Nutr.*, **35**, 968–972

PISCIOTTA, A. V. (1969) Agranulocytosis induced by certain phenothiazine derivatives. *J. Am. Med. Assoc.*, **208**, 1862–1868

REIGER, W., BRADY, J. P. and WEISBERG, E. (1978) Hematologic changes in anorexia nervosa. *Am. J. Psychiatry*, **135**, 984–985

SILVERMAN, J. A. (1974) Anorexia nervosa: clinical observations in a successful treatment plan. *J. Pediatr.*, **84**, 68–73

SMITH, R. L. R. and SPIVAK, J. L. (1985) Marrow cell necrosis in anorexia nervosa and involuntary starvation. *Br. J. Haematol.*, **60**, 525–530

TAVASSOLI, M., EASTLAND, D. T., YAM, L. T., NEIMAN, R. S. and FINKEL, H. (1976) Gelatinous transformation of bone marrow in prolonged self-induced starvation. *Scand. J. Haematol.*, **16**, 311–319

WADE, S., BLEIBERG, F., MOSSE, A., LUBETZKI, J., FLAVIGNY, H., CHAPVIS, P. *et al.* (1985) Thymulin (Zn-facteur thymique serique) activity in anorexia nervosa patients. *Am. J. Clin. Nutr.*, **42**, 275–278

WARREN, M. P. and VANDE WIELE, R. L. (1973) Clinical and metabolic features of anorexia nervosa. *Am. J. Obstet. Gynecol.*, **117**, 435–449

WYATT, R. J., FARRELL, M., BERRY, P. L., FORRISTAL, J., MALONEY, M. J. and WEST, C. D. (1982) Reduced alternative complement pathway control protein levels in anorexia nervosa: response to parenteral alimentation. *Am. J. Clin. Nutr.*, **35**, 973–980

Chapter 10

Renal function and electrolytes

Renal function

Blood urea concentrations are usually normal or only slightly elevated in anorectics (Russell and Bruce, 1966; Warren and Vande Wiele, 1973; Kanis et al., 1974; Halmi and Falk, 1981). We measured blood urea and creatinine concentrations in 137 patients in our series and found a moderately raised blood urea in 22 (16%). However, the serum creatinine level was raised in only one purgative addict with a blood urea of 31.6 mmol/l and severe hypokalaemic alkalosis. The majority view is that, unless the levels are exceptionally high, any uraemia is due to pre-renal factors such as dehydration and increased protein catabolism.

In some patients dehydration may only be shown in retrospect by a drop in the haemoglobin concentration and haematocrit during the early days of treatment. Mild dehydration is difficult to detect clinically and may have a number of causes. It is uncommon for anorectics deliberately to restrict their fluid intake but many will lose water through vomiting, purgation or diuretic abuse. Another factor may be failure of the kidneys to conserve water.

Impaired water diuresis

Defects in both urinary concentration and dilution in anorexia nervosa have been known for many years. However, the impaired water diuresis in patients with this disease was not systematically investigated until Russell and Bruce (1966) tested the ability of anorectics to produce dilute urine after a water load. Twelve patients were studied, along with five patients with affective disorders who acted as controls. Diuresis was impaired in five of the anorectics, particularly when they were kept standing throughout the test. Neither body weight nor whether or not oedema was present correlated with the response, but impaired diuresis was found only in those who had been ill for more than 3 years. However, the degree of reduced water excretion did correlate with the glomerular filtration rate, as measured by the creatinine clearance test. After re-feeding, three of the patients showed some improvement in their ability to handle a water load, but full recovery took several months. One patient with impaired diuresis during the day passed a large amount of urine at night. It was thought that the most likely explanation was that the excretion of water, but not that of sodium or potassium, was facilitated by recumbency. Impaired diuresis is probably not uncommon in anorectics, for nocturia was a symptom in one-quarter of our patients.

Aperia, Broberger and Fohlin (1978) compared renal function in 12 young anorectics with that of five healthy teenagers of comparable age and height. All the patients' plasma electrolyte levels and serum protein concentrations were within the normal range. The glomerular filtration rate and renal plasma flow were determined by the clearance of inulin and para-aminohippuric acid respectively. Urinary concentrating capacity was measured by recording the maximal urine osmolality after 17 hours without food or water, before and after the administration of vasopressin. Both the glomerular filtration rate and the clearance of para-aminohippuric acid were generally reduced in the anorectics. However, the reduction of the glomerular filtration rate was out of proportion to the reduction in the renal plasma flow, as shown by a significantly lower filtration fraction in the anorectics compared with the controls. Indirect evidence suggested that the low filtration fraction could be attributed to reduced water permeability of the glomerular capillary. The urinary concentrating capacity following fluid deprivation was moderately depressed both before and after the administration of vasopressin, suggesting that the defect was of renal rather than of central origin.

In another study Boag et al. (1985) measured plasma creatinine concentration, urinary creatinine excretion and creatinine clearance in 10 anorectics before and after treatment. Urinary creatinine excretion and clearance were diminished in every case. After re-feeding and an increase in weight, nine patients showed significant falls in plasma creatinine levels and increases in creatinine clearance, even when adjustments were made for body weight and surface area. The patient who did not show these changes had gained only 4% in body weight. Boag et al. suggested that renal vasoconstriction and mild hypovolaemia might be responsible for the diminished ability by these patients to clear water through their kidneys.

Secretion of vasopressin

An alternative explanation for these reversible renal abnormalities is that there is some hypothalamic–pituitary dysfunction in these patients resulting in deficient or inappropriate secretion of the antidiuretic hormone, arginine vasopressin. Mecklenburg et al. (1974) measured urine osmolality after 15 hours of water deprivation in five anorectics and found that, although it was consistently greater than that of their plasma, the administration of exogenous vasopressin led to a further increase in the urine osmolality. This finding, which is compatible with partial diabetes insipidus, was confirmed by Vigersky et al. (1977).

Gold et al. (1983) pointed out that abnormal secretion of vasopressin cannot be inferred from urine osmolality alone, and carried out direct measurements of plasma and cerebrospinal fluid vasopressin in four anorectics and eight age-matched controls. Abnormal osmoregulation in response to intravenous hypertonic saline was found in all four patients. Although one patient had a simple deficiency of vasopressin secretion, the more common abnormality was erratic fluctuations in plasma vasopressin levels that bore no apparent relationship to changes in the plasma sodium concentration. Both defects took some months to disappear after weight restoration, and were accompanied by abnormalities in the levels of the hormone in the cerebrospinal fluid. All their patients had significantly increased urinary output but none had hypokalaemia, hypercalcaemia or any other recognized cause of nephrogenic diabetes insipidus.

Renal calculi

The only symptom commonly referable to the urinary tract is nocturia, but on rare occasions a patient may display symptoms and signs of renal calculi. Berkman (1948) noted that renal stones had been found in a number of cases and attributed this to a combination of reduced fluid intake and excess urinary calcium due to osteoporosis. One of the anorectics reported by Elkington and Huth (1959) was a woman who had been ill for at least 5 years and presented with dysuria and frank haematuria. Intravenous pyelography revealed a large calculus in her right kidney, but she refused to allow the stone to be removed. This patient had recurrent hypokalaemic alkalosis, hyponatraemia and hypermagnesaemia due to the ingestion of large quantities of magnesium hydroxide, and died suddenly at the age of 34.

A more recent and happier account is that provided by Silber and Kass (1984) who described a 17-year-old anorectic with severe abdominal pain, dysuria and haematuria. Cystoscopy and retrograde pyelography confirmed nephrolithiasis. The patient was managed conservatively and subsequently passed calcium oxalate stones. The authors concluded that a history of high oxalate consumption and diminished fluid intake, compounded by self-induced vomiting and purgative abuse, was sufficient to explain the calculi formation. They could not, however, rule out an underlying metabolic abnormality since she systematically sabotaged attempts to collect a 24-hour urine specimen. Finally, Bruch (1971) described a fatal case of anorexia nervosa in which excessive consumption of milk and vitamin D led to extensive nephrocalcinosis.

Electrolytes

Electrolyte disturbances are rare in those who lose weight by dieting alone, but are not uncommon in vomiters and purgers. They are likely to be particularly severe in patients taking laxatives over a long period. A reduced dietary intake combined with excessive losses of sodium, potassium, chloride and hydrogen ions from the stomach or large bowel may eventually lead to a metabolic alkalosis and potassium depletion. Dehydration, salt loss and consequent hypovolaemia activate the renin–angiotensin–aldosterone system and secondary aldosteronism, while aiding sodium conservation, will promote further loss of potassium from the kidneys. The taking of oral diuretics to increase the weight loss or to combat oedema will further exacerbate the situation. Incidentally, the oedema which is sometimes found in an untreated patient or during re-feeding has never been satisfactorily explained; the most likely cause is a high salt intake in an individual with an overactive renin–angiotensin–aldosterone system.

The reported incidence of abnormal electrolytes in anorexia nervosa has varied widely, possibly because the subjects studied included differing proportions of vomiters and purgers. In some studies all the patients had normal levels (Kanis et al., 1974; Halmi and Falk, 1981). Warren and Vande Wiele (1973) reported abnormal electrolytes in only one of their 42 anorectics, the exception being a woman who had been vomiting repeatedly. By contrast, Elkinton and Huth (1959) studied 20 patients and found a hypochloraemic alkalosis at some time in seven. This was usually associated with self-induced vomiting and occurred only in those who had lost at least 25% of their normal body weight. Hypokalaemia was present in four of their cases. Similarly, Warren and Steinberg (1979) found a hypokalaemic alkalosis in four of their seven patients. In two it was associated with U waves on the electrocardiogram.

Primary respiratory alkalosis often coincided with the metabolic alkalosis in their patients, occasionally resulting in a dangerous elevation of the blood pH.

The prevalence of these electrolyte abnormalities in clinical practice is not clear from these reports. Serum electrolytes were measured in 129 patients under our care. Fifteen (12%) had serum potassium levels below 3.5 mmol/l, but none had hypochloraemia and only four had elevated serum bicarbonate concentrations. In most of these patients the serum potassium level lay between 3.0 and 3.4 mmol/l and was usually corrected by giving oral potassium supplements. Two purgative addicts presented with severe hypokalaemic alkalosis and required intravenous therapy to restore their electrolytes to normal. Our only patient with hyponatraemia was one of these purgers with evidence of renal damage.

Potassium depletion

Potassium deficiency should be suspected if an anorectic complains of muscle weakness, paraesthesiae, polydipsia or nocturia. Hypokalaemia, which is not necessarily accompanied by hypochloraemia or an elevated serum bicarbonate level, will confirm the diagnosis. Wolff *et al.* (1968) carried out detailed metabolic studies in nine psychiatrically disturbed women suffering from the effects of anorexia nervosa, vomiting and the abuse of diuretics and purgatives. Each had more than one source of electrolyte depletion and each deliberately concealed at least one of them. All were potassium-depleted, and in all but one sodium depletion was also evident. During exacerbations plasma renin concentration was raised, secretion rate and plasma concentration of aldosterone were increased, and the metabolic clearance of aldosterone was diminished. The authors suggested that in combined sodium and potassium deficiency, conservation of sodium may be relatively more effective than that of potassium and that multiple routes of electrolyte loss prevent effective homeostasis.

Although severe potassium depletion appears to be uncommon in anorectics, it is potentially dangerous and can result in renal impairment, profound muscular weakness and life-threatening cardiac arrhythmias. Relman and Schwartz (1956) were among the first to draw attention to the nephropathy caused by potassium depletion in man. Their five subjects consisted of two emaciated middle-aged males with chronic diarrhoea due to intestinal disease, and three females who had abused laxatives over a long period. No specific mention was made of anorexia nervosa, but it may be relevant that one 25-year-old woman had lost some 14 kg in weight over the previous two years. All the patients were hypokalaemic, but only one had a mildly elevated serum bicarbonate concentration and the urinary excretion of potassium in all five patients was less than 10 mmol/day. The blood urea nitrogen levels were not significantly increased but all the patients had evidence of both glomerular and tubular dysfunction. The renal clearances of inulin, urea and creatinine were reduced and none produced a more concentrated urine in response to vasopressin. Renal biopsies in three of their patients showed diffuse non-specific degeneration of the tubular epithelium. The characteristic vacuolation of the convoluted tubules, which had been previously reported in potassium-depleted rats and human subjects, was seen only in one case. There were no abnormalities of the glomeruli or blood vessels to explain the apparent defects in glomerular function. Potassium replacement produced total healing of these lesions in one patient and marked improvement in another; renal function returned to normal in four patients after a delay of several weeks. The authors pointed out that a normal level of potassium in the serum does not necessarily rule out potassium depletion, and that the functional consequences may persist long after the serum potassium level has been restored to normal.

Four years later Wigley (1960) drew attention to the relationship between hypokalaemia and renal impairment in anorexia nervosa. He reviewed the existing literature and added three cases of his own, making a total of 20. Many of these patients were alkalotic in addition to their hypokalaemia, some were hyponatraemic, and 11 had evidence of renal dysfunction. All his patients complained of generalized muscle weakness. Marked tubular vacuolation was found on renal biopsy and confirmed at autopsy in one patient who succumbed to a pneumonia. No less than five of the 20 patients he described had died by the time his paper was published.

Magnesium deficiency

Magnesium deficiency is a rare finding in this disease, but life-threatening hypomagnesaemia was described by Fonseca and Havard (1985) in a 32-year-old female anorectic with a long history of diuretic and purgative abuse. On admission to hospital because of weakness, paraesthesiae and tetany she was found to have a marked proximal muscle weakness and gross emaciation. Abnormal laboratory findings included anaemia, moderate uraemia, hypokalaemia and hypocalcaemia. In spite of blood transfusion and intravenous therapy with potassium chloride and calcium gluconate the plasma concentrations of potassium and calcium remained low. The patient's presenting symptoms persisted and she went on to develop congestive cardiac failure. Normal serum parathyroid hormone and 25-hydroxyvitamin D concentrations excluded hypoparathyroidism and vitamin D deficiency as the cause of the hypocalcaemia. She was, however, found to have a low plasma magnesium level of 0.56 mmol/l. The intravenous administration of magnesium sulphate over a period of 4 days was followed by the rapid resolution of the electrolyte disturbances, and then the cardiac failure. Over the next 6 months her plasma magnesium concentration remained within the normal range and the size and functioning of her heart remained normal.

Magnesium deficiency may result from a diminished dietary intake or excessive losses through the gastrointestinal tract or kidneys. All these factors were probably operating in this patient for she was described as cachectic on admission and had a long history of laxative and diuretic abuse. Many diuretics, particularly the loop-blocking compounds such as frusemide, increase magnesium excretion in the urine by a direct action on the renal tubules and indirectly by activating the renin–angiotensin–aldosterone system. Aldosterone promotes the loss of both potassium and magnesium from kidneys and colon, the former more rapidly than the latter. Thus hypokalaemia is often evident in weeks but the consequent hypomagnesaemia may not be detectable for years. This may explain why hypokalaemia is not uncommon in vomiters and purgers but hypomagnesaemia is rare. The reversible cardiac failure and muscular weakness in this woman were almost certainly due to the combined effects of potassium and magnesium deficiency on the myocardium and skeletal muscle.

Calcium and phosphate metabolism

Hypocalcaemia is uncommon in anorexia nervosa and, in most cases, is probably due to vitamin D deficiency. We measured serum calcium, phosphate, and alkaline phosphatase concentrations in 129 patients in our series and found hypocalcaemia in

Table 10.1 Biochemical osteomalacia in an 18-year-old female

	Serum albumin (g/l)	Serum calcium (total) (mmol/l)	Serum ionized calcium (mmol/l)	Serum phosphate (mmol/l)	Serum alkaline phosphatase (IU/l)
On admission	39	2.03	1.01	0.78	223
Calciferol for 10 days	39	2.47	1.21	1.41	83
Normal range	32–50	2.20–2.62	1.07–1.27	0.80–1.45	25–85

seven (5.4%). The lowest level of 1.60 mmol/l was in a chronic purgative abuser, but her serum phosphate level was elevated at 2.51 mmol/l and she had evidence of severe renal damage caused by potassium depletion. In only one of the other six patients was the hypocalcaemia accompanied by a subnormal serum phosphate level and a raised alkaline phosphatase concentration. This 18-year-old female had been ill for less than one year but was grossly emaciated on admission. It was clear from these findings that she had osteomalacia and her response to oral calciferol in a dose of 75 µg daily for 10 days is shown in *Table 10.1*. In the remaining five patients the hypocalcaemia disappeared when they were given oral vitamin D supplements and gained weight.

Fonseca *et al.* (1985) studied 16 anorectics and found that the median serum concentration of 25-hydroxyvitamin D was significantly lower than in their control subjects, and that the patients with anorexia nervosa had markedly diminished mineral bone density. They suggested that lack of vitamin D may contribute to the pathogenesis of osteopenia in patients with this disorder.

A contrary view was expressed by Rigotti *et al.* (1984) who found normal blood levels of 25-hydroxyvitamin D and 1,25-dihydroxyvitamin D in 18 anorectic women who had been ill for at least 3 years. Bone densitometry by direct photon absorptiometry showed that these patients had a significantly lower cortical bone density than the 28 normal controls. The bone density correlated moderately with age, weight loss and duration of illness. All their patients had normal serum calcium, phosphate and albumin levels and the serum alkaline phosphatase concentration was raised only in one patient who had recently sustained a vertebral compression fracture. However, the calculated calcium intake was remarkably low, and only two patients had an intake of more than 300 mg/day. Bone biopsy in one patient provided no evidence of osteomalacia but showed thinned trabeculae and minimal osteoblast activity, consistent with osteoporosis. They concluded that the osteopenia in their patients may have been caused by a combination of oestrogen deficiency, dietary calcium deficiency, and excessive glucocorticoid secretion.

Szmukler *et al.* (1985) also investigated premature loss of bone in chronic anorexia nervosa. They studied five patients who had had the disease for over 10 years. Four of their cases had radiological evidence of vertebral crush fractures, but none of the bone biopsies showed evidence of osteomalacia. Nevertheless, one patient did have a low serum calcium of 2.0 mmol/l and a raised serum alkaline phosphatase of 266 IU/l, so that vitamin D deficiency may have contributed to the bone disease in this individual.

A rare cause of hypocalcaemia in anorexia nervosa is magnesium deficiency. In the patient with refractory hypocalcaemia and hypomagnesaemia described by Fonseca and Havard (1985), the plasma calcium concentration failed to rise into the normal range despite the intravenous administration of large amounts of calcium gluconate for 10 days. The rapid correction of the hypocalcaemia following magnesium replacement was accompanied by a substantial rise in the level of parathyroid hormone in the serum. Anast *et al.* (1976) and others have shown that the secretion of parathyroid hormone in response to hypocalcaemia is impaired in the presence of hypomagnesaemia, and that the low magnesium level and related hypocalcaemia can be corrected by surprisingly small amounts of intravenous magnesium.

Low serum phosphate levels on their own are rarely seen. We found only two such cases in our series and both these patients denied self-induced vomiting or purgative abuse. However, Sheridan and Collins (1983) have reported a near-fatal case of hypophosphataemia in an anorectic who not only abused laxatives, but consumed little in the way of phosphorus-containing foods such as meat, milk products or eggs. The initial biochemical evaluation revealed nothing abnormal, but her serum phosphate level was 0.9 mmol/l, close to the lower end of the normal range. As the patient refused food she was tube-fed with a high calorie liquid diet. She responded by taking a large dose of laxative stolen from the medicine trolley. Following this episode the serum phosphate concentration fell to 0.13 mmol/l. The patient was transferred to the intensive care unit, but the expected cardiorespiratory failure did not develop, and instead abdominal ileus occurred. Phosphate supplements were given intravenously and later orally once the ileus had resolved. Within a relatively short time both her weight and serum phosphate level were satisfactory. The authors argued that, in states of phosphorus depletion, refeeding without sufficient extra phosphate results in the transfer of phosphorus to muscle and liver cells to initiate anabolic activity. This causes a rapid fall in the serum phosphate concentration and hence a potentially dangerous reduction in the supply of phosphorus to vital organs such as the heart and brain.

Summary

Defects in urinary concentration and dilution are not uncommon in patients with anorexia nervosa, particularly if they have been ill for more than 2 years. Whether these are due to hypovolaemia, renal vasoconstriction or to some hypothalamic abnormality in the control of vasopressin secretion is still uncertain. Apart from nocturia they cause little in the way of symptoms and are reversible following weight gain. The only common electrolyte disturbance is potassium depletion which is found mainly in vomiters and purgers and may have serious effects on kidneys, skeletal muscle and cardiac function. Hypocalcaemia is occasionally seen and is probably due to deficiency of vitamin D in the diet.

References

ANAST, C. S., WINNACKER, J. I., FORTE, I. R. and BURNS, T. W. (1976) Impaired release of parathyroid hormone in magnesium deficiency. *J. Clin. Endocrinol. Metab.*, **42**, 707–717

APERIA, A., BROBERGER, O. and FOHLIN, L. (1978) Renal function in anorexia nervosa. *Acta Paediatr. Scand.*, **67**, 219–224

BERKMAN, J. M. (1948) Anorexia nervosa, anterior-pituitary insufficiency, Simmond's cachexia, and Sheehan's disease. *Postgrad. Med.*, **3**, 237–246

BOAG, F., WEERAKOON, J., GINSBURG, J., HAVARD, C. W. H. and DANDONA, P. (1985) Diminished creatinine clearance in anorexia nervosa: reversal with weight gain. *J. Clin. Pathol.*, **38**, 60–63

BRUCH H. (1971) Death in anorexia nervosa. *Psychosom. Med.*, **33**, 135–144

ELKINTON, J. R. and HUTH, E. J. (1959) Body fluid abnormalities in anorexia nervosa and undernutrition. *Metabolism*, **8**, 376–403

FONSECA, V. and HAVARD, C. W. H. (1985) Electrolyte disturbances and cardiac failure with hypomagnesaemia in anorexia nervosa. *Br. Med. J.*, **291**, 1680–1682

FONSECA, V., HOULDER, S., THOMAS, M., D'SOUZA, V., WAKELING, A. and DANDONA, P. (1985) Osteopenia in women with anorexia nervosa. *N. Engl. J. Med.*, **313**, 326

GOLD, P. W., KAYE, W., ROBERTSON, G. L. and EBERT, M. (1983) Abnormalities in plasma and cerebrospinal-fluid arginine vasopressin in patients with anorexia nervosa. *N. Engl. J. Med.*, **308**, 1117–1123

HALMI, K. A. and FALK, J. R. (1981) Common physiological changes in anorexia nervosa. *Int. J. Eating Disorders*, **1**, 16–27

KANIS, J. A., BROWN, P., FITZPATRICK, K., HIBBERT, D. J., HORN, D. B., NAIRN, I. M. et al. (1974) Anorexia nervosa: a clinical, psychiatric and laboratory study. *Q. J. Med.*, **67**, 321–328

MECKLENBERG, R. S., LORIAUX, D. L., THOMPSON, R. H., ANDERSEN, A. E. and LIPSETT, M. B. (1974) Hypothalamic dysfunction in patients with anorexia nervosa. *Medicine*, **53**, 147–159

RELMAN, A. S. and SCHWARTZ, W. B. (1956) The nephropathy of potassium depletion: a clinical and pathological entity. *N. Engl. J. Med.*, **255**, 195–203

RIGOTTI, N. A., NUSSBAUM, S. R., HERZOG, D. B. and NEER, R. M. (1984) Osteoporosis in women with anorexia nervosa. *N. Engl. J. Med.*, **311**, 1601–1606

RUSSELL, G. F. M. and BRUCE, J. T. (1966) Impaired water diuresis in patients with anorexia nervosa. *Am. J. Med.*, **40**, 38–48

SHERIDAN, P. H. and COLLINS, M. (1983) Potentially life-threatening hypophosphatemia in anorexia nervosa. *J. Adolesc. Health Care*, **4**, 44–46

SILBER, T. J. and KASS, E. J. (1984) Anorexia nervosa and nephrolithiasis. *J. Adolesc. Health Care*, **5**, 50–52

SZMUKLER, G. I., BROWN, S. W., PARSONS, V. and DARBY, A. (1985) Premature loss of bone in chronic anorexia nervosa. *Br. Med. J.*, **290**, 26–27

VIGERSKY, R. A., ANDERSEN, A. E., THOMPSON, R. H. and LORIAUX, D. L. (1977) Hypothalamic dysfunction in secondary amenorrhea associated with simple weight loss. *N. Engl. J. Med.*, **297**, 1141–1145

WARREN, M. P. and VANDE WIELE, R. L. (1973) Clinical and metabolic features of anorexia nervosa. *Am. J. Obstet. Gynecol.*, **117**, 435–449

WARREN, S. E. and STEINBERG, S. M. (1979) Acid-base and electrolyte disturbances in anorexia nervosa. *Am. J. Psychiatry*, **136**, 415–418

WIGLEY, R. D. (1960) Potassium deficiency in anorexia nervosa with reference to renal tubular vacuolation. *Br. Med. J.*, ii, 110–113

WOLFF, H. P., VECSEI, P., KRUCK, F., ROSCHER, S., BROWN, J. J., DUSTERDIECK, G. O. et al. (1968) Psychiatric disturbance leading to potassium depletion, raised plasma-renin concentration, and secondary hyperaldosteronism. *Lancet*, i, 257–261

Chapter 11

The endocrine system

Anorexia nervosa is associated with many abnormalities of endocrine and hypothalamic function. Thermoregulation is often faulty and partial diabetes insipidus is not uncommon, particularly in the more severe cases. Most of the endocrine disorders appear to be due to abnormalities in the hypothalamic regulation of anterior pituitary function and the consequent effect upon its target organs. Whether these changes are caused by primary hypothalamic disease or are secondary to the weight loss alone is still uncertain, but similar disturbances have been reported in adults with protein-calorie malnutrition and, to a lesser extent, in mildly obese women who have lost weight on reducing diets (Vigersky *et al.*, 1977).

On the other hand, the rare occurrence of typical anorexia nervosa in teenagers and young adults with hypothalamic tumours, the fact that the amenorrhoea often precedes other manifestations of the disease, and the presence of some of these abnormalities in patients of normal weight suffering from endogenous depression, are in favour of a primary hypothalamic disorder. It is conceivable that psychological stresses in a vulnerable individual produce reversible biochemical changes in the hypothalamus which trigger off these disturbances in the first place, and they are then perpetuated by the resulting loss of weight.

Gonadal function

Early cessation of menstruation has long been recognized as one of the cardinal features of this disorder. The amenorrhoea may precede, follow or coincide with the abnormal eating behaviour and loss of weight. In about one-half of the patients in our series it occurred before there was any appreciable weight loss. This makes it unlikely that the amenorrhoea is the result of starvation.

Hypothalamic dysfunction

Numerous studies have shown that the hypothalamus and pituitary are involved in this lack of periods. Serum gonadotrophins are low and the response to the administration of gonadotrophin-releasing hormone is often blunted (Boyar *et al.*, 1974; Sherman, Halmi and Zamudio, 1975). The nocturnal increase in serum luteinizing hormone (LH) levels which occurs in healthy postpubertal girls is absent, and the pattern of LH secretion resembles that seen in prepubertal children. Beumont, Pimstone and Vinik (1976) reported that the LH response to gonadotrophin-releasing hormone improved as their patients gained weight, but did not return to normal until they had been within 10% of their calculated optimum weight for several months. Katz *et al.* (1978), in a similar study, found that those women who showed both weight gain and normalization of the adult circadian LH secretory pattern were also symptomatically improved in other respects, but the return of the menses did not show a simple relationship to weight, fatness or maturity of the LH pattern.

Marshall and Fraser (1971) found that the plasma LH levels were low in underweight anorectics and failed to rise after the administration of clomiphene citrate. When there was a return to normal weight the LH levels rose normally in response to this drug, and this was often accompanied by a return of regular menstrual cycles. Clomiphene is sometimes of value in triggering off menstruation when the amenorrhoea persists, despite maintaining normal body weight for several months.

Ovarian function

Plasma oestradiol levels are low in severely underweight patients but return to normal once the weight exceeds about 80% of the optimum for age and height. There is a marked increase in the metabolic conversion of oestradiol to 2-hydroxyoestrone with a compensatory decrease in oestriol. Whether these changes in oestradiol metabolism are related to changes in body fat or to hepatic dysfunction is unknown (Fishman, Boyar and Hellman, 1975). The plasma progesterone levels are also low.

The widespread use of pelvic ultrasonography in the investigation of ovulatory disorders has led to the discovery of multifollicular ovarian cysts in anorectics who are putting on weight (Adams *et al.*, 1985; Treasure *et al.*, 1985). These changes in the morphology of the ovaries resemble those seen in the prepubertal girl and probably represent a normal ovarian response to the hypothalamic disturbance of gonadotrophin control. Unlike the polycystic ovary syndrome (Stein–Leventhal syndrome) this condition is not associated with hirsutism, and the cysts are said to disappear when the patients start normal ovulatory cycles.

Gonadal function in the male

Anorexia nervosa is so uncommon in the male that few endocrine studies have been carried out. Those that have been performed show similar hypothalamic disturbances to those seen in the female. Rapid and complete loss of libido and sexual activity usually occurs within a few weeks of the onset of dieting.

Hall, Delahunt and Ellis (1984) studied nine male patients and found that the plasma testosterone in the two patients in whom it was measured was very low. Libido and normal sexual activity did not return until their weight was nearly normal for their age and height. Four patients were fully investigated at follow-up. Three adult males had recovered to at least 90% of their normal weight for more than 6 months and had normal LH and follicle-stimulating hormone (FSH) responses to gonadotrophin-releasing hormone. Two had normal plasma testosterone levels, but the level in one 22-year-old man was still subnormal. One teenager who had early pubertal changes at the time of onset of the disease, had not resumed growth or advanced in puberty despite a high calorie intake and a satisfactory weight for height for over one year. His plasma testosterone level and LH response to gonadotrophin-releasing hormone were still at prepubertal levels, but he had normal thyroid function and no evidence of growth hormone deficiency.

Prolactin secretion

Serum prolactin levels usually fall within the normal range in anorectics unless the patient is taking dopamine antagonists such as chlorpromazine or metoclopramide (Isaacs, 1979). The rise in prolactin levels following an intravenous bolus of thyrotrophin-releasing hormone (TRH) is a crude test of pituitary prolactin reserve. Isaacs studied the response to TRH in 11 patients before and after weight gain, and found that the mean level at 20 minutes after the injection of TRH was considerably lower than normal. When the test was repeated after weight gain the response was completely normal.

We have measured basal serum prolactin levels and the response to the intravenous injection of 200 µg of TRH in 12 female anorectics, both before and after regaining at least 90% of their calculated optimum weight. The basal serum prolactin level was 210 ± 33 mu/l (mean $\pm$ s.e.m.), the normal range for our laboratory being less than 400 mu/l. There was a sevenfold rise in the mean prolactin level 20 minutes after the TRH was given. The levels rose even higher after the patients had regained their lost weight, but this was probably due to the fact that they had been treated with dopamine antagonists and were still receiving them up to the time of the test (*Figure 11.1*).

There seems to be little evidence that prolactin secretion is significantly altered in anorexia nervosa or plays any part in the menstrual disturbances, but the reduced

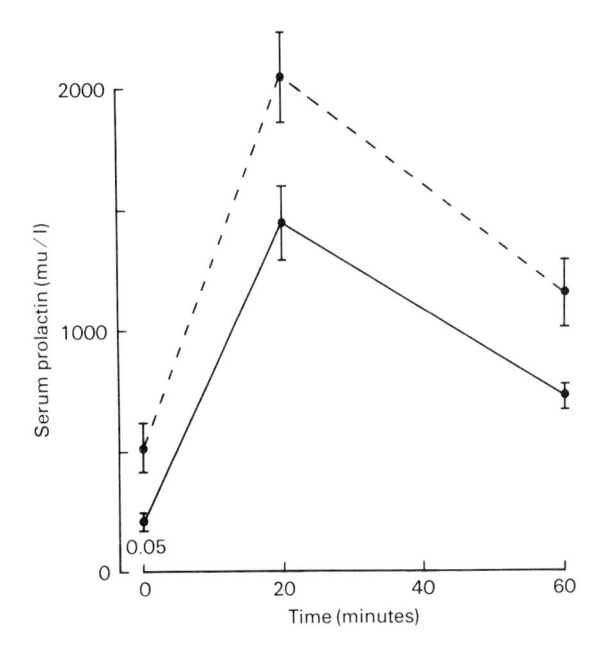

Figure 11.1 Serum prolactin levels (mean $\pm$ s.e.m.) during a TRH test in 12 patients before treatment and after weight gain on neuroleptic drugs. An intravenous injection of 200 µg of TRH was given at zero time. *P* values are shown when significant. ●——● Before treatment; ●– –● after treatment

response to TRH noted by Isaacs and others is compatible with the theory of Barry and Klawans (1976) that there is dopamine overactivity in the hypothalamus in this disease.

Thyroid function

Early claims that patients with anorexia nervosa were suffering from hypothyroidism were based on the common complaints of cold intolerance, constipation, bradycardia, dry skin and diminished sweating, supported by the almost universal finding of low basal metabolic rates. Later studies, using radioiodine uptake tests and measurement of the serum protein-bound iodine, failed to demonstrate any consistent abnormalities of thyroid function. It was not until reliable radioimmunoassays for serum thyroxine (T4), tri-iodothyronine (T3) and thyrotrophin (TSH) became available that any progress was made.

Low T3 syndrome

Many investigators have now confirmed the presence of consistently low serum T3 levels in anorexia nervosa, together with low or low normal serum T4 levels and normal TSH concentrations (Miyai *et al.*, 1975; Moshang *et al.*, 1975; Travaglini *et al.*, 1976; Boyar *et al.*, 1977; Croxson and Ibbertson, 1977; Moore and Mills, 1979). These abnormalities are typical of the 'low T3 syndrome' found in patients with severe non-thyroidal illness, in fasted obese subjects and in protein-calorie malnutrition. Common to all these conditions is undernutrition so that the low T3 syndrome may be an adaptive process to limit catabolism.

The low serum T3 levels are probably the result of decreased conversion of thyroxine to tri-iodothyronine in the liver, and increased production of its metabolically inactive isomer, reverse T3 (rT3). Elevated rT3 levels have been found in some anorectics and returned to normal after the patients had gained weight (Leslie *et al.*, 1978). Several studies have shown that there is an inverse correlation between the serum T3 levels and the severity of the weight loss in this disease.

Moore and Mills (1979) measured serum T3 and T4 levels in 33 patients who had lost at least 25% of their original weight, 21 patients with primary hypothyroidism and 25 healthy women. The serum T3 levels in the anorectics were significantly lower than those in the controls and patients with myxoedema, while serum T4 levels were higher than those in the patients with primary hypothyroidism but lower than those in the control group. There was a significant rise in the serum T3 levels in 18 anorectics after a 25% weight gain, the increase being directly proportional to the rate of weight gain rather than the gain itself. In 14 patients the hormone levels were monitored weekly during inpatient treatment. The majority showed a gradual rise in the serum T3 levels to the high normal range during refeeding, but in four patients there was a distinct and sustained overshoot accompanied by signs of a temporary and self-limiting hyperthyroid state. All four were putting on weight rapidly beforehand, but during the period of high serum T3 levels the rate of weight gain slowed down and they complained of heat intolerance and showed signs of peripheral vasodilatation. The authors pointed out that there was a danger of demoralization and false accusations about occult vomiting or hiding of food, unless the cause of the temporary slowing down in weight gain was appreciated and explained to the patient and all those concerned with her care.

The evidence that these low serum T3 levels in anorexia nervosa are indicative of a tissue hormone deficiency is largely indirect. Fowler, Manim and Ikram (1972) were among the first to show that the Achilles reflex half-relaxation time was prolonged in this disease, as it is in hypothyroid patients. This was confirmed by Croxson and Ibbertson (1977) who found that it was prolonged in two-thirds of their 38 patients. The administration of 40 µg of tri-iodothyronine daily for four weeks to 11 anorectics, before significant weight gain had occurred, restored the Achilles reflex half-relaxation time to normal. In addition, there are changes in the hepatic metabolism of steroids in this condition which are also found in hypothyroid patients. These include a significant decrease in the metabolic clearance of cortisol, a prolongation of the cortisol half-life in the plasma, a significant decrease in the urinary and rosterone/etiocholanolone ratio and an increased urinary tetrahydrocortisol/tetrahydrocortisone ratio. All these abnormalities are corrected by the administration of tri-iodothyronine (Bradlow et al., 1976; Boyar et al., 1977).

Hypothalamic dysfunction

In patients with primary hypothyroidism the subnormal levels of thyroid hormones in the blood provoke a compensatory rise in pituitary TSH secretion. This does not occur in the low T3 syndrome found in anorexia nervosa. Quite apart from the alteration in the peripheral metabolism of T3 and T4 there must be some additional defect in the central control of TSH secretion in these patients. Although basal serum TSH levels are normal there is a delayed response to the stimulatory effect of TRH in anorectics which is similar to that seen in patients with hypothalamic disease (Miyai et al., 1975; Leslie et al., 1978; Norris, O'Malley and Palmer, 1985).

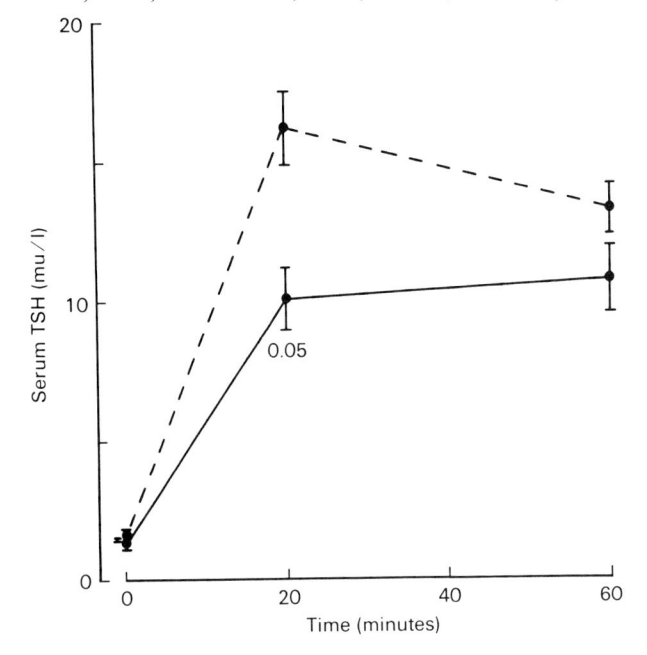

Figure 11.2 Serum TSH levels (mean ± s.e.m.) during a TRH test in 18 patients before treatment and after weight gain on neuroleptic drugs. An intravenous injection of 200 µg of TRH was given at zero time. P values are shown when significant. ●——● Before treatment; ●---● after treatment

We have carried out TRH tests in 18 anorectics, both before treatment and after they had regained at least 80% of their optimum weight on dopamine antagonists. On admission their serum T4 level (mean ± s.e.m.) was in the low normal range at 77.8 ± 4.2 nmol/l. Only four patients had subnormal T4 levels. Serum TSH levels were measured at 0, 20 and 60 minutes after the injection. After satisfactory weight gain, and while still taking dopamine antagonists, there was a significantly greater rise at 20 minutes (*Figure 11.2*). Dopamine is the neurotransmitter secreted by the hypothalamus which inhibits the release of prolactin and TSH from the anterior pituitary. The blunted response to TRH which is seen in anorexia nervosa provides further indirect evidence to support the hypothesis that there is dopamine overactivity in the hypothalamus in this disorder.

Adrenal function

The old idea that adrenocortical function is subnormal in this disorder has long since been discredited, but it is only relatively recently that it has become apparent that the opposite state of affairs exists. As tests became more sophisticated it was found that patients with anorexia nervosa tended to have higher than normal levels of cortisol in plasma and urine, although the normal circadian variation in cortisol secretion was preserved and their cortisol production rates fell within the normal range for healthy adults (Kanis *et al.*, 1974; Boyar *et al.*, 1977).

Boyar *et al.* (1977) found normal cortisol production rates in their patients, but the rate of cortisol metabolism was slowed down. They suggested that this was due to hypothyroidism and was sufficient to explain the elevated plasma cortisol levels. Walsh *et al.* (1981) were not satisfied with this explanation and measured cortisol production before and after recovery in 10 anorectics. Their major finding was that, as patients with anorexia nervosa recover, their rate of cortisol secretion decreases. They suggested that adrenal secretory activity is increased in this condition, and that the elevation of the plasma cortisol levels reflects not only a slowing of cortisol metabolism, but also a rise in cortisol production. Doerr *et al.* (1980) reached a similar conclusion on the basis of measurements of the 24-hour profile of plasma cortisol, and the lack of normal suppression of the pituitary–adrenal axis by dexamethasone.

Inappropriate ACTH secretion

Resistance of the hypothalamic–pituitary–adrenal axis to suppression by exogenous glucorticoids is a major feature of pituitary-dependent Cushing's syndrome and is thought to be a measure of altered corticotrophin-releasing hormone regulation in the hypothalamus. Several studies have shown that plasma cortisol levels are not suppressed normally by dexamethasone in a significant proportion of anorectic patients (Walsh *et al.*, 1978; Doerr *et al.*, 1980; Gerner and Gwirtsman, 1981). However, this abnormality is not confined to anorexia nervosa for it has been found in patients of normal weight with endogenous depression (Carroll, Curtis and Mendels, 1976; Gold *et al.*, 1986a), and in some cases of bulimia (Hudson *et al.*, 1983). It is also present, along with other evidence of adrenocortical overactivity, in adults with severe protein-calorie malnutrition (Smith, Bledsoe and Chhetri, 1975).

Gold *et al.* (1986b) examined plasma ACTH and cortisol responses to an intravenous bolus of ovine corticotrophin-releasing hormone (CRH) in 15 anorectics, both before and after correction of weight loss. Initially the anorectics had marked hypercorticalism with impaired dexamethasone suppression but normal basal plasma ACTH levels. This was associated with a marked reduction in the plasma ACTH response to CRH. When these patients were studied 3–4 weeks after their body weight had been restored to normal, the hypercorticalism had resolved but the abnormal response to CRH was unchanged. However, 6 months later their responses were normal. This study included patients with bulimia whose weight was normal and they too had a normal response to CRH. The authors suggested that the hypercorticalism in their anorectics was due to an abnormality at or above the hypothalamus that caused hypersecretion of corticotrophin-releasing hormone.

A similar study carried out by Hotta *et al.* (1986) confirmed these results. In addition, they found that the mean concentration of immunoreactive CRH in the cerebrospinal fluid of seven patients was significantly higher than in their controls. The origin of CRH in the cerebrospinal fluid is unknown but it has been detected by radioimmunoassay in extrahypothalamic brain tissue such as amygdala, hippocampus, thalamus and cingulate cortex, as well as in the hypothalamic paraventricular nuclei. The authors suggested that the hypersecretion of CRH from extrahypothalamic as well as hypothalamic sites might play a part in the pathogenesis of anorexia nervosa.

Association with Cushing's syndrome

When we studied adrenocortical function in 29 anorectic patients some years ago we found elevated plasma and urinary 11-hydroxycorticoids in seven; in two emaciated females they were comparable to those found in severe Cushing's syndrome. In view of the recent findings of an increased secretion of corticotrophin-releasing hormone in anorexia nervosa this is not surprising, but the hypercorticalism in this disorder is usually less marked than that in pituitary-dependent Cushing's disease, is reversible on weight gain, and is not accompanied by any overt signs of cortisol excess.

There are, however, a few cases in the literature of the occurrence of both Cushing's syndrome and anorexia nervosa in the same individual. Black *et al.* (1965) were the first to draw attention to this association. Their patient developed Cushing's syndrome at the age of 14 and presented with the typical appearance of anorexia nervosa one year later. Marked redness of the cheeks, a high blood pressure and her previous appearance in a photograph suggested the diagnosis of adrenocortical overactivity, which was confirmed biochemically. She underwent bilateral adrenalectomy, and histology of the glands showed a prominent cortex with microadenomas. Her postoperative recovery was uneventful, and 10 months later her weight and appearance were normal and she had resumed menstruation.

In the case described by Katz *et al.* (1986) the presentation was somewhat different. At the age of 15 the patient developed anorexia nervosa and became preoccupied with her diet and weight. Fifteen months later she began to gain weight rapidly despite continuing and frantic efforts to diet. During the next 8 months there were rapid fluctuations in weight and fluid retention, and she began to binge with subsequent vomiting. There was little in her physical appearance to suggest adrenocortical overactivity and her blood pressure was only 100/60, but her morning plasma cortisol concentration and urinary free cortisol excretion were markedly elevated. At operation both adrenals were found to be enlarged. Two years later she noted increasing pigmentation and complained of frequent headaches, but a CT scan of her head was apparently normal. Later her plasma ACTH was found to be markedly elevated and skull tomograms now showed an enlarged sella turcica. Four years after her bilateral adrenalectomy the diagnosis of Cushing's disease was established when a pituitary adenoma was removed surgically. The authors suggested that the two conditions could be related, although not in a cause and effect way. They proposed that the pituitary adenoma was activated by the hypothalamically-mediated stimulation of the pituitary–adrenal axis found in anorexia nervosa, and eventually resulted in full-blown Cushing's disease.

In both the above cases there was a fairly close temporal relationship between the onset of the two diseases. In the only other case that we could find in the literature, symptoms of hypercorticalism appeared some 12 years after the onset and persistence of classical anorexia nervosa (Kontula *et al.*, 1984). This patient also had an ACTH-secreting pituitary tumour.

Mineralocorticoid excess

Activation of the renin–angiotensin–aldosterone system in vomiters and purgers as a result of dehydration and electrolyte loss has already been discussed in the previous chapter. Secondary aldosteronism could be responsible for the pitting oedema of the legs which is not uncommonly seen in untreated patients, and which may appear for the first time on refeeding. Pasternack (1970) described a 29-year-old female anorectic with a long history of surreptitious vomiting and unexplained diarrhoea. On admission she had severe hypokalaemia, hyponatraemia, hypochloraemia and a metabolic alkalosis. Urinary aldosterone levels were increased on two occasions. Plasma renin activity was grossly elevated and was not suppressed by a high sodium intake. Renal biopsy revealed hyperplasia of the juxtaglomerular complex, narrowing of medium-sized and small arteries, focal interstitial fibrosis and hyalinization of glomeruli in areas corresponding to the vascular alterations. The angiopathy was not confined to the kidneys as biopsy of the quadriceps muscle showed thickened arteries and arterioles. Over the next 2 years she complained of pain in her right foot, and was readmitted because of threatening gangrene of the right big toe. Angiography showed complete occlusion of the right popliteal artery and narrowing of the femoral arteries and their branches on both sides. Pasternack suggested that high renin–angiotensin activity, by causing long-standing vasoconstriction, had given rise to these vascular abnormalities.

Growth hormone and carbohydrate metabolism

Normally the plasma glucose level rises after a carbohydrate meal and insulin is secreted, the secretion of growth hormone being suppressed. When the plasma glucose level returns to its fasting level about 2 hours later the secretion of insulin ceases and the output of glucagon and growth hormone rise, with a corresponding increase in their plasma levels. Glucagon increases gluconeogenesis from amino acids, and the lipolytic action of growth hormone on the fat depots releases free fatty acids as alternative fuel. The preferential uptake and oxidation of free fatty acids by muscle has a glucose-sparing effect, and together these two mechanisms usually prevent the plasma glucose concentration falling to dangerous levels between meals or during a prolonged fast.

Hypoglycaemia

Symptomatic hypoglycaemia is uncommon in anorexia nervosa despite the marked reduction in carbohydrate intake. Nevertheless, despite the lack of symptoms the fasting plasma glucose level is often at or below the lower limit of the fasting range for healthy individuals. In 91 anorectics in our series the fasting plasma glucose level was only 3.9 ± 0.06 mmol/l (mean ± s.e.m.); two-thirds of these patients had levels which were below our normal fasting range of 4.2–6.5 mmol/l.

There are several accounts of coma and even death resulting from severe spontaneous hypoglycaemia in this disease (Zalin and Lant, 1984; Ratcliffe and Bevan, 1985). One of our earlier cases, who was later discovered to have a hypothalamic astrocytoma, lapsed into hypoglycaemic coma one night and died 2 weeks later without regaining consciousness (Lewin, Mattingly and Millis, 1972). It is possible that unrecognized hypoglycaemia may account for some of the cases of sudden death in anorectics which have been reported in the past.

Landon *et al.* (1966) found that patients with anorexia nervosa showed an increased sensitivity to exogenous insulin, and this has been confirmed by others. In our experience, as little as two units of subcutaneous insulin after meals may produce hypoglycaemia in these patients before they start to put on weight. This enhanced sensitivity to insulin is probably due to an increased number of insulin receptors in the tissues. Wachslicht-Rodbard *et al.* (1979) studied insulin binding to erythrocytes and monocytes in eight anorectics and 17 controls. Their untreated patients showed increased binding to receptors on the circulating cells, which reverted to normal after weight gain. This abnormality was due to an increased number of receptors per cell, with little or no change in receptor affinity. The authors pointed out that a similar increase in insulin binding was found in other conditions of enhanced sensitivity to insulin such as growth hormone and glucocorticoid deficiency.

A more recent study by Zuniga-Guajardo, Garfinkel and Zinman (1986), using the glucose clamp technique, found increased insulin sensitivity with decreased basal insulin levels and increased clearance in nine female anorectics. The authors suggested that these were adaptive changes to calorie restriction and were reversible on refeeding and weight gain.

Growth hormone

Hypoglycaemia normally provokes a rise in growth hormone secretion. The low fasting plasma glucose levels in anorectics probably account for the elevated fasting growth hormone levels which are sometimes found (Landon *et al.*, 1966; Brown *et al.*, 1977; Hurd, Palumbo and Gharib, 1977). Even when the fasting levels are normal, glucose loading often results in a paradoxical rise in serum growth hormone concentrations instead of the usual suppression (Kanis *et al.*, 1974; Casper, Davis and Pandey, 1977). These abnormalities are associated with a diabetic type of glucose tolerance curve, the plasma glucose level failing to return to the fasting state within 2 hours.

Similar changes in response to a glucose load have been reported in gross malnutrition from other causes (Alvarez *et al.*, 1972). The same pattern of growth hormone secretion and impaired glucose tolerance is also seen in acromegaly, but in anorexia nervosa there are no clinical signs of growth hormone excess and this is probably due to defective formation of somatomedins in the liver (Rappaport, Prevot and Czernichow, 1980). The lipolytic effects of growth hormone, in contrast to the

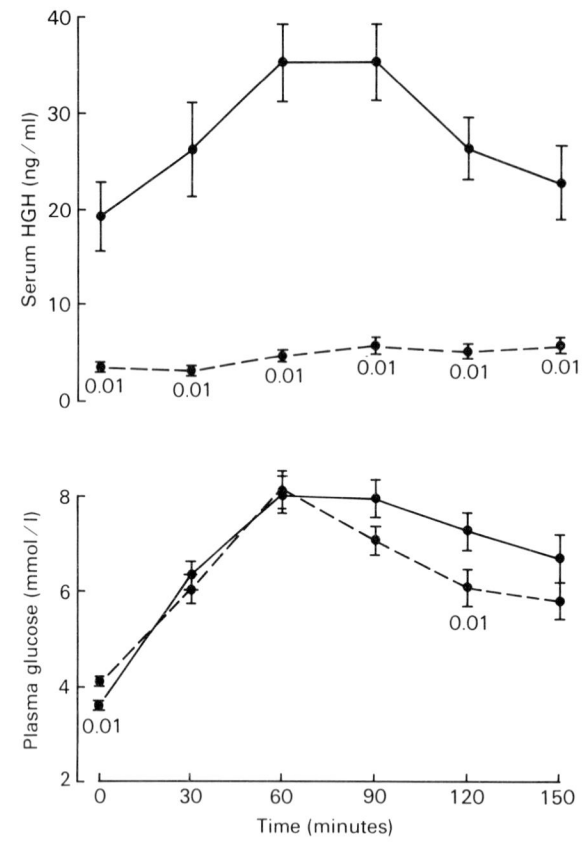

Figure 11.3 Oral glucose tolerance tests in 36 untreated anorectics. Twenty patients in group I, (●——●) had grossly abnormal serum growth hormone levels (mean ± s.e.m.) throughout the test and showed a paradoxical rise. The 16 patients in group II (●--●) had normal fasting levels but did not suppress normally. Impaired glucose tolerance was present in both groups of patients. P values are shown when significant

effects on growth and protein synthesis, are not dependent on somatomedin generation.

We measured serum growth hormone levels during an oral glucose tolerance test in 36 anorectic patients. They were given 75 g of glucose in the morning after an overnight fast. In 20 subjects the growth hormone levels were not suppressed and showed a marked paradoxical rise; one-half of the patients in this group had elevated fasting levels. In the remaining 16 patients the fasting growth hormone levels were normal but there was little evidence of suppression and the levels tended to rise rather than fall after the first hour. Impaired glucose tolerance was present in both groups but was more marked in those with grossly abnormal growth hormone responses (*Figure 11.3*). Previous reports had suggested that the abnormality in growth hormone secretion might be related to the severity of weight loss. However, we found no significant difference between the two groups with regard to age, duration of illness, actual body weight or the degree of weight loss. The mean weight loss, expressed as a percentage of their optimum weight, was around 30% in both groups.

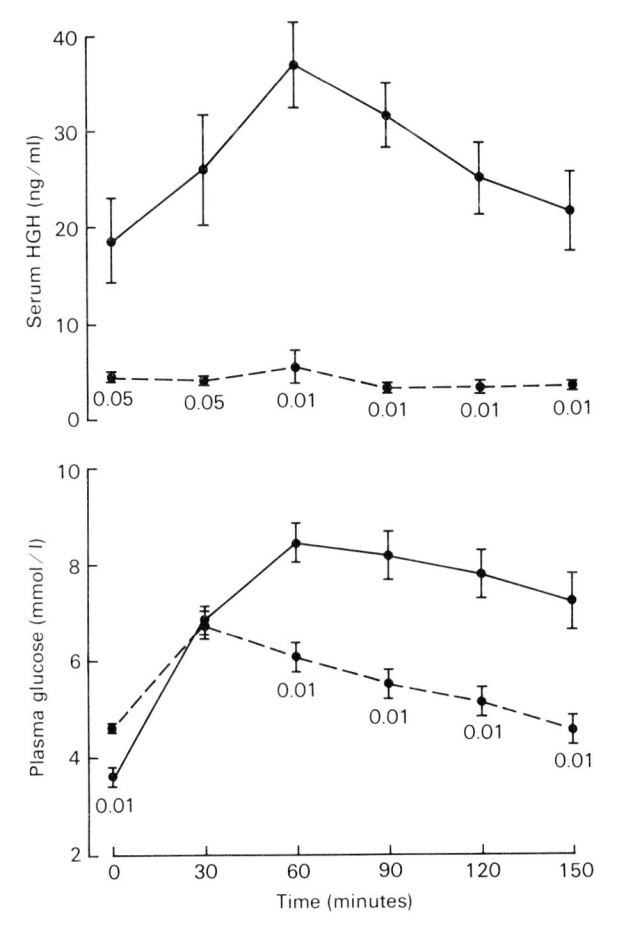

Figure 11.4 Oral glucose tolerance tests in 17 patients with grossly abnormal growth hormone curves, before treatment and after weight gain on neuroleptic drugs. Serum growth hormone and plasma glucose levels (mean ± s.e.m.) returned to normal after treatment. P values are shown when significant. ●——● Before treatment; ●---● after treatment

The only significant difference between the groups was in the mean fasting plasma glucose concentration which was lower in those with the grossly abnormal responses ($P < 0.01$). Fifteen of the 20 patients in this group had fasting plasma glucose levels below our normal range.

Abnormal growth hormone secretion following a glucose load is probably a reflection of the nutritional state of the patient at the time the test is performed. It is a measure of the hypothalamic response to starvation and helps to protect the anorectic from death by hypoglycaemia.

The studies were repeated in 17 of the 20 patients with grossly abnormal responses 5–6 weeks later, when they had regained at least 80% of their calculated optimum weight on insulin and neuroleptic drugs. The growth hormone responses were now normal and the impaired glucose tolerance had disappeared (*Figure 11.4*).

Insulin secretion

The fasting levels of insulin in patients with anorexia nervosa usually fall within the normal range, but Ratcliffe and Bevan (1985) were unable to detect any C peptide or insulin in the blood of their two patients with severe hypoglycaemia. On the other hand, the impaired glucose tolerance which occurs during an oral or intravenous glucose tolerance test is accompanied by a sustained rise in serum insulin levels (Crisp, Ellis and Lowy, 1967; Kanis et al., 1974). Similar changes are seen in normal adults after only 5 days on a low carbohydrate diet (Hales and Randle, 1963).

The impaired glucose tolerance in these situations is probably due to a combination of the lipolytic effect of increased growth hormone secretion leading to higher levels of free fatty acids in the blood, and increased gluconeogenesis from amino acids as a result of excess cortisol or glucagon. If this hypothesis is correct then the sustained secretion of insulin is a physiological response to the raised plasma glucose levels.

Blickle et al. (1984) studied 26 anorectics and found a paradoxical rise in growth hormone secretion in all of them during an intravenous glucose tolerance test, but were unable to demonstrate any consistent increase in glucagon secretion. Unlike other workers, they found a significantly diminished insulin response to glucose loading in their patients, and concluded that the regulation of fuel supply during chronic starvation depended mainly on changes in insulin and growth hormone secretion.

The impaired glucose tolerance in anorexia nervosa is readily reversible on weight gain, as was demonstrated in our patients. Crisp, Ellis and Lowy (1967) found that the sustained insulin response persisted to some extent in two patients who were studied after one year's full recovery, but this has not been confirmed by others.

The pineal gland

Pinealomas were found in some of the cases described in Chapter 2 who presented as anorexia nervosa and were later found to have hypothalamic or midbrain tumours. A major product of the pineal gland, melatonin, is known to influence carbohydrate metabolism and reproductive activity in animals. Its secretion may be abnormal in those who are depressed, and may be reduced in those taking neuroleptic medication of the type which may be of benefit in anorexia nervosa. Melatonin has been a difficult substance to assay and only a few studies have been carried out on its plasma concentrations in anorectics. Garfinkel and Garner (1982) cited an apparently unpublished report by Brown et al. All six patients showed the expected nocturnal rise in plasma melatonin levels. Dalery et al. (1985) investigated eight cases and confirmed that the normal circadian rhythm was maintained. The mean peak plasma level, however, was higher than in a control group of depressed patients. Melatonin secretion was also enhanced in the 14 anorectics studied by Ferrari et al. (1987).

Thanks to the assistance of Dr Josephine Arendt and Christine Franey of the University of Surrey we have been able to study the 24-hour plasma melatonin profiles in 10 anorectics and in three patients with bulimia nervosa. The assay technique used was that of Fraser et al. (1983). The peak levels in all subjects occurred during the night, and in eight of the anorectics were higher than those usually observed. On the other hand, the peak levels in the bulimics were not elevated.

Summary

The various endocrine disorders that are found in anorexia nervosa appear to be due to a combination of hypothalamic dysfunction and alterations in the peripheral metabolism of insulin, steroids and thyroid hormones. Similar changes have been reported in protein-calorie malnutrition and in other wasting diseases. While many of these disturbances can be attributed to the nutritional state of the patient, this cannot apply to the secondary amenorrhoea which is a cardinal feature of this condition and often precedes any significant loss of weight. The neuroendocrine abnormalities improve on refeeding, but it may be many months after achieving normal weight before they disappear completely. Only when menstruation is fully established can one be reasonably sure that the patient will not relapse. A primary hypothalamic dysfunction in anorexia nervosa cannot be excluded on the evidence available at present.

References

ADAMS, J., FRANKS, S., POLSON, D. W., MASON, H. D., ABDULWAHID, N., TUCKER, M. *et al.* (1985) Multifollicular ovaries: clinical and endocrine features and response to pulsatile gonadotrophin-releasing hormone. *Lancet*, ii, 1375–1381

ALVAREZ, L. C., DIMAS, C. O., CASTRO, A., ROSSMAN, L. G., VANDERLAAN, E. F. and VANDERLAAN, W. P. (1972) Growth hormone in malnutrition. *J. Clin. Endocrinol. Metab.*, 34, 400–409

BARRY, V. C. and KLAWANS, H. L. (1976) On the role of dopamine in the pathophysiology of anorexia nervosa. *J. Neural Transm.*, 38, 107–122

BEUMONT, P. J. V., PIMSTONE, G. B. L. and VINIK, A. I. (1976) Body weight and the pituitary response to hypothalamic releasing hormones in patients with anorexia nervosa. *J. Clin. Endocrinol. Metab.*, 43, 487–495

BLACK, M. M., HALL, R., KAY, D. W. K. and KILBORN, J. R. (1965) Anorexia nervosa in Cushing's syndrome. *J. Clin. Endocrinol. Metab.*, 25, 1030–1034

BLICKLE, J. F., REVILLE, P., STEPHAN, F., MEYER, P., DEMANGEAT, C. and SAPIN, R. (1984) The role of insulin, glucagon and growth hormone in the regulation of plasma glucose and free fatty acid levels in anorexia nervosa. *Horm. metab. Res.*, 16, 336–340

BOYAR, R. M., HELLMAN, L. D., ROFFWARG, H., KATZ, J., ZUMOFF, B., O'CONNOR, J. *et al.* (1977) Cortisol secretion and metabolism in anorexia nervosa. *N. Engl. J. Med.*, 296, 190–193

BOYAR, R. M., KATZ, J., FINKELSTEIN, J. W., KAPEN, S., WEINER, H., WETZMAN, E. D. *et al.* (1974) Anorexia nervosa: immaturity of the 24-hour luteinizing hormone secretory pattern. *N. Eng. J. Med.*, 291, 861–865

BRADLOW, H. L., BOYAR, R. M., O'CONNOR, J., ZUMOFF, B. and HELLMAN, L. (1976) Hypothyroid-like alterations in testosterone metabolism in anorexia nervosa. *J. Clin. Endocrinol. Metab.*, 43, 571–574

BROWN, G. M., GARFINKEL, P. E., JEUNIEWIC, N., MOLDOFSKY, H. and STANCER, H. C. (1977) Endocrine profiles in anorexia nervosa. In *Anorexia Nervosa*, edited by R. A. Vigersky, pp. 125–127. New York: Raven Press.

CARROLL, B. J., CURTIS, G. C. and MENDELS, J. (1976) Neuroendocrine regulation in depression. *Arch. Gen. Psychiatry*, 33, 1039–1044

CASPER, R. C., DAVIS, J. M. and PANDEY, G. N. (1977) The effect of nutritional status and weight changes on hypothalamic function tests in anorexia nervosa. In *Anorexia Nervosa*, edited by R. A. Vigersky, pp. 138–143. New York: Raven Press

CRISP, A. H., ELLIS, J. and LOWY, C. (1967) Insulin response to a rapid intravenous injection of dextrose in patients with anorexia nervosa and obesity. *Postgrad. Med. J.*, 43, 97–102

CROXSON, M. S. and IBBERTSON, H. K. (1977) Low serum triiodothyronine and hypothyroidism in anorexia nervosa. *J. Clin. Endocrinol. Metab.*, 44, 167–174

DALERY, J., CLAUSTRAT, B., BRUN, J., TERRA, J. L., CHAZOT, G. and DE VILLARD, R. (1985) Profils journaliers de

la melatonie, du cortisol et des gonadotrophines chez 8 adolescentes porteuses d'une anorexie mentale. *Encephale*, **11**, 25–28
DOERR, P., FICHTER, M., PIRKE, K. M. and LUND, R. (1980) Relationship between weight gain and hypothalamic–pituitary–adrenal function in patients with anorexia nervosa. *J. Steroid Biochem.*, **13**, 529–537
FERRARI, E., BOSSOLO, P. A., FOPPA, S., COMIS, S., FRASCHINI, F. and BRAMBILLA, F. (1987) Melatonin and pituitary-gonadal secretion in disorders of eating behaviour. *Proc. IV Colloquium of the European Pineal Study Group*, p. 49 (abstract)
FISHMAN, J., BOYAR, R. M. and HELLMAN, L. (1975) Influence of body weight on oestradiol metabolism in young women. *J. Clin. Endocrinol. Metab.*, **41**, 989–991
FOWLER, P. B. S., MANIM, S. O. and IKRAM, H. (1972) Prolonged ankle reflex in anorexia nervosa. *Lancet*, ii, 307–308
FRASER, S., COWEN, P., FRANKLIN, M., FRANEY, C. and ARENDT, J. (1983) Direct radioimmunoassay for melatonin in plasma. *Clin. Chem.*, **29**, 396–397
GARFINKEL, P. E. and GARNER, D. M. (1982) Hypothalamic–pituitary function in anorexia nervosa. In *Anorexia Nervosa: a Multidimensional Perspective*, pp. 80–81. New York: Brunner/Mazel
GERNER, R. H. and GWIRTSMAN, H. E. (1981) Abnormalities of dexamethasone suppression test and urinary MHPG in anorexia nervosa. *Am. J. Psychiatry*, **138**, 650–653
GOLD, P. W., LORIAUX, D. L., ROY, A., KLING, M. A., CALABRESE, J. R., KELLNER, C. H. *et al.* (1986a) Response to corticotrophin-releasing hormone in the hypercortisolism of depression and Cushing's disease. *N. Engl. J. Med.*, **314**, 1329–1335
GOLD, P. W., GWIRTSMAN, H., AVGERINOS, P., NIEMAN, L. K., GALLUCCI, W., KAYE, W. *et al.* (1986b) Abnormal hypothalamic–pituitary–adrenal function in anorexia nervosa: pathophysiologic mechanisms in underweight and weight-corrected patients. *N. Engl. J. Med.*, **314**, 1335–1342
HALES, C. N. and RANDLE, P. J. (1963) Effects of low-carbohydrate diet and diabetes mellitus on plasma concentrations of glucose, non-esterified fatty acid, and insulin during oral glucose tolerance tests. *Lancet*, i, 790–794
HALL, A., DELAHUNT, J. W. and ELLIS, P. M. (1984) Anorexia nervosa in the male: clinical features and follow-up of nine patients. *J. Psychiat. Res.*, **19**, 315–321
HOTTA, M., SHIBASAKI, T., MASUDA, A., IMAKI, T., DEMURA, H., LING, N. *et al.* (1986) The responses of plasma adrenocorticotrophin and cortisol to corticotrophin-releasing hormone (CRH) and cerebrospinal fluid immunoreactive CRH in anorexia nervosa patients. *J. Clin. Endocrinol. Metab.*, **62**, 319–324
HUDSON, J. I., POPE, H. G., JONAS, J. M., LAFFER, P. S., HUDSON, M. S. and MELBY, J. C. (1983) Hypothalamic–pituitary–adrenal axis hyperactivity in bulimia. *Psychiatry. Res.*, **8**, 111–117
HURD, H. P., PALUMBO, P. J. and GHARIB, H. (1977) Hypothalamic–endocrine dysfunction in anorexia nervosa. *Mayo Clin. Proc.*, **52**, 711–716
ISAACS, A. J. (1979) Endocrinology. In *Anorexia Nervosa*, edited by P. Dally and J. Gomez, p. 196. London: Heinemann
KANIS, J. A., BROWN, P., FITZPATRICK, K., HIBBERT, D. J., HORN, D. B., NAIRN, I. M. *et al.* (1974) Anorexia nervosa: a clinical, psychiatric and laboratory study. *Quart. J. Med.*, **43**, 321–338
KATZ, J. L., BOYAR, R. M., ROFFWARG, H., HELLMAN, L. and WEINER, H. (1978) Weight and circadian luteinizing hormone secretory pattern in anorexia nervosa. *Psychosomatic. Med.*, **40**, 549–567
KATZ, J. L., WEINER, H., KREAM, J. and ZUMOFF, B. (1986) Cushing's disease in a young woman with anorexia nervosa: pathophysiological implications *Can. J. Psychiatry*, **31**, 861–864
KONTULA, K., MUSTAJOKI, P., PAETAU, A. and PELKONEN, R. (1984) Development of Cushing's disease in a patient with anorexia nervosa. *J. Endocrinol. Invest.*, **7**, 35–40
LANDON, J., GREENWOOD, F. C., STAMP, C. B. and WYNN, V. (1966) The plasma sugar, free fatty acid, cortisol and growth hormone response to insulin, and the comparison of this procedure with other tests of pituitary and adrenal function. II. In patients with hypothalamic or pituitary dysfunction or anorexia nervosa. *J. Clin. Invest.*, **45**, 437–449
LESLIE, R. D. G., ISAACS, A. J., GOMEZ, J., RAGGATT, P. R. and BAYLISS, R. (1978) Hypothalamo–pituitary–thyroid function in anorexia nervosa: influence of weight gain. *Br. Med. J.*, ii, 526–528
LEWIN, K., MATTINGLY, D. and MILLIS, R. R. (1972) Anorexia nervosa associated with hypothalamic tumour. *Br. Med. J.*, ii, 629–630
MARSHALL, J. C. and FRASER, T. R. (1971) Amenorrhoea in anorexia nervosa: assessment and treatment with clomiphene citrate. *Br. Med. J.*, **4**, 590–592

MIYAI, K., YAMAMOTO, T., AZUKIZAWA, M., ISHIBASHI, K. and KUMAHARA, Y. (1975) Serum thyroid hormones and thyrotrophin in anorexia nervosa. *J. Clin. Endocrinol. Metab.*, **40**, 334–338

MOORE, R. and MILLS, I. H. (1979) Serum T3 and T4 levels in patients with anorexia nervosa showing transient hyperthyroidism during weight gain. *Clin. Endocrinol.*, **10**, 443–449

MOSHANG, T., PARKS, J. S., BAKER, L., VAIDYA, V., UTIGER, R. D., BONGIOVANNI, A. M. *et al.* (1975) Low serum triiodothyronine in patients with anorexia nervosa. *J. Clin. Endocrinol. Metab.*, **40**, 470–472

NORRIS, P. D., O'MALLEY, B. P. and PALMER, R. L. (1985) The TRH test in bulimia and anorexia nervosa: a controlled study. *J. Psychiatr. Res.*, **19**, 215–219

PASTERNACK, A. (1970) Anorexia nervosa, secondary aldosteronism and angiopathy. *Acta Med. Scand.*, **187**, 139–143

RAPPAPORT, R., PREVOT, C. and CZERNICHOW, P. (1980) Somatomedin activity and growth hormone secretion: changes related to body weight in anorexia nervosa. *Acta Paediatr. Scand.*, **69**, 37–41

RATCLIFFE, P. J. and BEVAN, J. S. (1985) Severe hypoglycaemia and sudden death in anorexia nervosa. *Psychol. Med.*, **15**, 679–681

SHERMAN, B. M., HALMI, K. A. and ZAMUDIO, R. (1975) LH and FSH response to gonadotrophin-releasing hormone in anorexia nervosa: effect of nutritional rehabilitation. *J. Clin. Endocrinol. Metab.*, **41**, 135–142

SMITH, S. R., BLEDSOE, T. and CHHETRI, M. K. (1975) Cortisol metabolism and the pituitary-adrenal axis in adults with protein-calorie malnutrition. *J. Clin. Endocrinol. Metab.*, **40**, 43–52

TRAVAGLINI, P., BECK-PECCOZ, P., FERRARI, C., AMBROSI, B., PARACCHI, A., SEVERGNINI, A. *et al.* (1976) Some aspects of hypothalamic–pituitary function in patients with anorexia nervosa. *Acta Endocrinol.*, **81**, 252–262

TREASURE, J. L., GORDON, P. A. L., KING, E. A., WHEELER, M. and RUSSELL, G. F. M. (1985) Cystic ovaries: a phase of anorexia nervosa. *Lancet*, ii, 1379–1384

VIGERSKY, R. A., ANDERSEN, A. E., THOMPSON, R. H. and LORIAUX, D. L. (1977) Hypothalamic dysfunction in secondary amenorrhoea associated with simple weight loss. *N. Engl. J. Med.*, **297**, 1141–1145

WACHSLICHT-RODBARD, H., GROSS, H. A., RODBARD, D., EBERT, M. H. and ROTH, J. (1979) Increased insulin binding to erythrocytes in anorexia nervosa. *N. Engl. J. Med.*, **300**, 882–887

WALSH, B. T., KATZ, J. L., LEVIN, J., KREAM, J., FUKUSHIMA, D. K., HELLMAN, L. D. *et al.* (1978) Adrenal activity in anorexia nervosa. *Psychosom. Med.*, **40**, 499–506

WALSH, B. T., KATZ, J. L., LEVIN, J., KREAM, J., FUKUSHIMA, D. K., WEINER, H. *et al.* (1981) The production rate of cortisol declines during recovery from anorexia nervosa. *J. Clin. Endocrinol. Metab.*, **53**, 203–205

ZALIN, A. M. and LANT, A. F. (1984) Anorexia nervosa presenting as reversible hypoglycaemic coma. *J. Roy. Soc. Med.*, **77**, 193–195

ZUNIGA-GUAJARDO, S., GARFINKEL, P. E. and ZINMAN, B. (1986) Changes in insulin sensitivity and clearance in anorexia nervosa. *Metabolism*, **35**, 1096–1100

Chapter 12

Cholesterol and carotene

Hypercholesterolaemia and hypercarotenaemia appear to be benign concomitants of anorexia nervosa, and do not lead to serious complications. Their causes are not known, but both can be of diagnostic importance in difficult cases since they do not occur in other wasting diseases such as malignancy and intestinal malabsorption.

Hypercholesterolaemia

Crisp (1965) and Klinefelter (1965) are usually accredited with first drawing attention to hypercholesterolaemia in anorexia nervosa. The former, in presenting his findings in 30 anorectics, noted that most had serum cholesterol levels of 10.4 mmol/l or over. He regarded a diet rich in cheese as playing a major role. As the patients recovered, their serum cholesterol concentrations fell. Klinefelter, having encountered two patients in whom serum cholesterol levels were unexpectedly raised, reviewed the records of 98 patients seen at the Johns Hopkins hospital over the previous 30 years. Hypercholesterolaemia had been recorded in approximately one-third of the cases, particularly the younger ones. There was no relationship between the cholesterol levels and the length of time the patients had been ill, nor was it possible to attribute hypercholesterolaemia to any particular diet. However, the last had been investigated in detail in only a few cases.

In contrast to the above, there are a number of more recent reports which suggest that hypercholesterolaemia is only rarely found in anorexia nervosa, and some have noted the presence of low serum cholesterol levels such as might be expected in other forms of starvation. Pops and Schwabe (1968) found raised serum cholesterol levels in only two of their 12 cases, and Robboy, Sato and Schwabe (1974) found none, but studied only four patients. Halmi and Fry (1974) and Halmi and Falk (1981) regarded hypercholesterolaemia as an uncommon finding in anorexia nervosa, and noted that some cases had low levels which increased with weight gain. Nevertheless, the majority opinion is that raised serum cholesterol levels are an important feature of the illness. Milner, McAnarney and Klish (1985), for example, found that one-third of their patients had elevated serum cholesterol concentrations. This was similar to our finding in 91 cases (Mattingly and Bhanji, 1982).

Although clinical features of hypothyroidism are lacking, it is well recognized that many anorectics have low basal metabolic rates and low serum T3 levels. However, it does not appear that the hypercholesterolaemia is related to thyroid deficiency (Crisp, Blendis and Pawan, 1968; Kanis et al., 1974; Hurd, Palumbo and Gharib, 1977;

Mordasini, Klose and Greten, 1978). Blendis and Crisp (1968) suggested that hypercholesterolaemia is associated with a feeding pattern which includes episodic carbohydrate binges, and that those with normal cholesterol levels tended to eat small, regular meals low in carbohydrate. This opinion was supported by Fabry and Tepperman (1970) who presented and discussed evidence that, in man and laboratory animals, less frequent meals tended to result in raised serum cholesterol levels. Halmi and Fry (1974) investigated seven bulimic anorectics and five who had never binged, but were unable to confirm that the serum cholesterol concentration was higher in the former group. We were not able to demonstrate any relationship between hypercholesterolaemia and vomiting or purging (Bhanji and Mattingly, 1981).

Cholesterol metabolism

Because of the failure to establish any clear connection between serum cholesterol level and dietary content or eating habits, interest has turned to abnormalities of cholesterol metabolism. Nestel (1974) carried out sterol balance studies in four female anorectics, three of whom had hypercholesterolaemia. Dietary intake studies showed that the patients consumed less cholesterol than did healthy people of comparable age. Measurements of faecal sterol and bile acid excretion revealed that the anorectics were retaining dietary cholesterol. In the patient who was reassessed after treatment, the serum cholesterol level had fallen, the excretion of bile acids had increased, and her sterol balance had changed to one of net excretion. The author concluded that the changes in serum cholesterol in anorectics could derive from starvation-induced reductions in bile acid excretion and cholesterol catabolism.

Mordasini, Klose and Greten (1978) examined 18 anorectics and found that 11 were hypercholesterolaemic, and that this was due to an increase in the cholesterol transported in the β-lipoproteins. Cholesterol concentrations in the high-density and in the very low-density lipoproteins were as expected in the normal population. A number of explanations for the type II hyperlipoproteinaemia, which did not correlate with the degree of weight loss, were considered. A diet low in calories was ruled out as isocaloric feeding had no effect; nor as noted above could hypothyroidism be held responsible. There was no evidence of increased low-density lipoprotein synthesis, but it was noted that delayed catabolism would be consistent with the findings of Nestel (1974). The view most favoured, however, was that the secondary type II hyperlipoproteinaemia of anorexia nervosa is the result of a dramatic mobilization of body fat to provide an energy source.

All the theories mentioned so far stress dietary factors, metabolic changes resulting from starvation, or both. Another view is that the raised serum cholesterol level in anorexia nervosa results from hypothalamic disturbances. Lupton *et al.* (1976) have cited evidence from animal experiments which suggests that stimulation of the lateral hypothalamus produces not only a rise in serum cholesterol, but also one associated with a transient reduction of bile secretion into the duodenum.

Hypercarotenaemia

Carotene is a yellow pigment found in many fruits and vegetables, particularly carrots, broccoli, spinach and pumpkins. After ingestion it is converted, mainly in the intestinal mucosa, to vitamin A. Hypercarotenaemia, like hypercholesterolaemia, can occur in a variety of conditions other than anorexia nervosa. These include a dietary excess of high-carotene food, diabetes mellitus, hypothyroidism, nephrosis, and various hyperlipaemias (Cohen, 1958). It is a benign condition, as only sufficient vitamin A is synthesized to meet the body's immediate requirements (Sharman, 1985). If the plasma levels of carotene are high enough, hypercarotenaemia manifests itself as a yellow-orange discoloration of the skin. This usually appears first on the palms, soles, and nasolabial folds, and is easily distinguished from jaundice as the sclera are not affected.

The presence of hypercarotenaemia in anorexia nervosa has been demonstrated in a number of studies. Warren and Vande Wiele (1973) found that five of their 13 cases had serum carotene concentrations greater than 3.6 µmol/l, and Hurd, Palumbo and Gharib (1977) found a similar proportion. However, Silverman (1974) and ourselves (Mattingly and Bhanji, 1982) reported incidences of over 50%.

Before Dally (1959) drew attention to a possible association between hypercarotenaemia and anorexia nervosa, there had been a number of reports of this condition in the literature. It is tempting to speculate that some of these patients were suffering from unrecognized anorexia nervosa. Greene and Blackford (1926) described six cases of diet-induced hypercarotenaemia, and were impressed by the fact that the reasons for dieting were the result of neurosis. However, all their cases were male and older than the typical anorectic, and weight loss was mentioned in only two. Levin and Silvers (1931) reported two female cases; one, aged 22 years, had been dieting for one year and had lost considerable weight before developing a 'nervous breakdown'. Unfortunately no comment was made regarding her periods. Anderson and Soley (1938) regarded hypercarotenaemia as harmful in itself, and noted that of the nine patients described in detail all but one had lost between 3.2 and 18.0 kg in weight. Most of the cases, who all appear to be male, complained of vague abdominal symptoms of the type encountered in anorexia nervosa. Cohen (1958) reported a case which he regarded as a unique example of an inborn failure to convert carotene to vitamin A. The patient was a 38-year-old female with a long history of yellow skin, but who claimed to take a normal diet. Points in favour of anorexia nervosa were loss of weight, a low basal metabolic rate, dry skin, moderate iron deficiency and leucopenia.

Dally (1959) reported the case of a 28-year-old woman with a 12-year history of anorexia nervosa, and yellowing of the skin for about one month. For the previous 10 years her diet had contained large amounts of fruit and cooked green vegetables. On investigation her serum carotene level was found to be raised at 4.3 µmol/l. The serum vitamin A concentration was also increased but the patient was not hypercholesterolaemic. Glucose tolerance and thyroid function tests were normal. She was treated with strict bed rest. Green vegetables were omitted from her diet and the intake of fresh fruit was restricted. The patient gained weight, but her pigmentation persisted and the serum carotene and vitamin A concentrations were still elevated. It was Dally's opinion that the patient's diet was not responsible for her hypercarotenaemia.

Crisp and Stonehill (1967) described a 23-year-old female chronic anorectic who, during a 6-month period, ate two large tins of spinach puree each day in addition to a diet consisting mainly of cheese, eggs, fruit and herring roes. Her skin became pigmented and she was found to have a grossly elevated serum carotene level of 54 µmol/l. In addition, her serum cholesterol concentration had increased during this period from 10.6 to 19.9 mmol/l. The adoption of a more normal diet resulted in the gradual disappearance of the pigmentation and falls in the serum levels of carotene and cholesterol to 4.6 µmol/l and 8.0 mmol/l, respectively. The authors disagreed with Dally, believing that the high dietary intake of carotene was responsible for the grossly elevated serum level. They also suggested that carotene and cholesterol metabolism might be interdependent.

Pops and Schwabe (1968) investigated twelve anorectics, nine of whom had serum carotene levels greater than 4.5 µmol/l. Eight of the patients were questioned about their diets, and all denied any excessive intake of carrots and other yellow vegetables and fruits. There was no mention of green vegetables, many of which have a high carotene content. Ten of the cases had normal serum cholesterol levels, and inspection of the data does not suggest any correlation between these and the levels of carotene. We have reviewed 74 anorectics, all of whom denied purgation or vomiting, in which estimations of both serum carotene and cholesterol levels had been carried out. The correlation coefficient between serum concentrations of carotene and cholesterol was positive and statistically significant ($r = +0.26$; $P < 0.05$).

Robboy, Sato and Schwabe (1974) compared the mean serum carotene, retinyl ester, retinol, and retinoic acid levels in 10 healthy, regularly menstruating females, 10 healthy postmenopausal women, 20 pregnant women, 24 oligomenorrhoeic females with infertility, 11 seriously ill cachectic patients of both sexes, and eight cases of anorexia nervosa. Statistically significant elevations of the mean serum carotene, retinyl ester, retinol and retinoic acid concentrations were found only in the anorectics. The serum carotene and retinyl ester levels were reduced in those with wasting due to physical disease. Only two of the anorectics admitted eating large amounts of carrots. Serum lipophoresis was normal in three out of five anorectics. The authors concluded that the changes seen in anorexia nervosa were due either to an increased consumption of carotene or vitamin A, or to an acquired and reversible defect in the utilization or metabolism of vitamin A. The latter view was supported by Curran-Celentano et al. (1985), but they did not consider the dietary intake of carotene to be important. A contrary opinion was expressed by Kemman, Pasquale and Skaf (1983) who reported on 10 women of normal weight with amenorrhoea due to hypothalamic dysfunction, and who had serum carotene levels ranging from 4.1 to 18.7 µmol/l. All were vegetarians who ate diets rich in raw vegetables. Modifying the patients' diets not only reduced the serum carotene levels, but also improved their menstrual status.

A final possible explanation of raised carotene levels is zinc deficiency, as this element may be involved in retinol metabolism because of its effect on the synthesis of retinol binding protein. Casper et al. (1980), however, were not able to demonstrate any significant correlation between the serum concentrations of zinc and carotene.

The relationship of serum carotene levels to subtypes of anorexia nervosa was investigated by us (Bhanji and Mattingly, 1981) and Schwabe et al. (1981). Both studies produced the novel finding that elevated concentrations were significantly less common among those who abuse purgatives or induce vomiting. Examination of our current data has enabled comparisons to be made between the mean serum carotene levels in 86 dieters, 27 vomiters or purgers, and seven cases of bulimia nervosa. The results are set out in *Figure 12.1*, and support our original impression. Four of those with bulimia nervosa, all of whom were close to their calculated optimum weight, had raised serum carotene concentrations and one had definite pigmentation. In contrast to our findings Curran-Celentano et al. (1985) reported that all their six anorectics who vomited and periodically binged had elevated serum carotene concentrations.

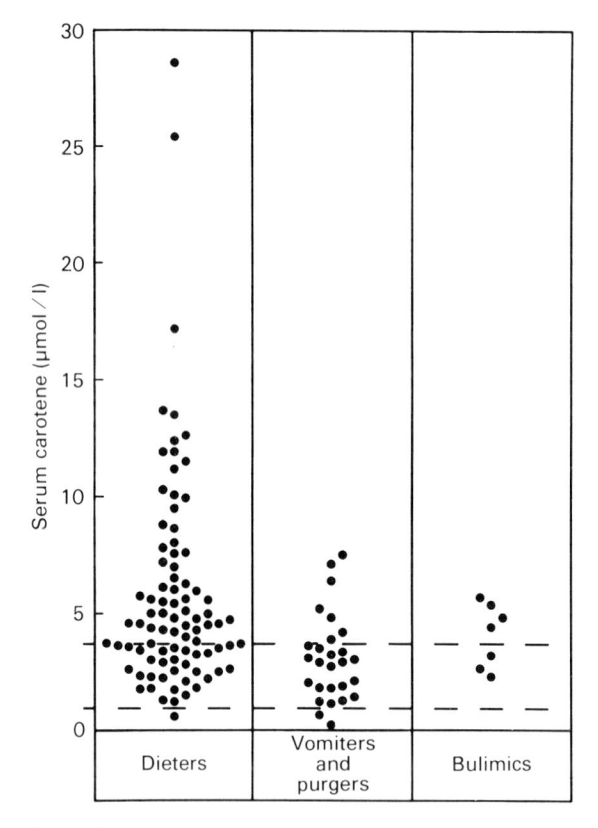

Figure 12.1 Serum carotene levels in 120 patients with eating disorders. The highest concentrations were found in anorectics who relied on dieting alone

Summary

Raised serum levels of both cholesterol and carotene are common findings in anorexia nervosa; they appear to be innocuous, but may assist in the diagnosis. Their causes are unknown, but many theories abound. In our view anorexia nervosa is the commonest cause of hypercarotenaemia in the UK today. The elevated carotene levels fall as the patient gains weight, but may not become normal for many months.

References

ANDERSON, H. H. and SOLEY, M. H. (1938) The effects of carotenemia on the function of the thyroid and the liver. *Am. J. Med. Sci.*, **195**, 313–318

BHANJI, S. and MATTINGLY, D. (1981) Anorexia nervosa: some observations on 'dieters' and 'vomiters and purgers', cholesterol and carotene. *Br. J. Psychiatry*, **139**, 238–241

BLENDIS, L. M. and CRISP, A. H. (1968) Serum cholesterol levels in anorexia nervosa. *Postgrad. Med. J.*, **44**, 327–330

CASPER, R. C., KIRSCHNER, B., SANDSTEAD, H. H., JACOB, R. A. and DAVIS, J. M. (1980) An evaluation of trace metals, vitamins, and taste function in anorexia nervosa. *Am. J. Clin. Nutr.*, **33**, 1801–1808

COHEN, H. (1958) Observations on carotenemia. *Ann. Intern. Med.*, **48**, 219–227

CRISP, A. H. (1965) Clinical and therapeutic aspects of anorexia nervosa—a study of 30 cases. *J. Psychosom. Res.*, **9**, 67–77

CRISP, A. H., BLENDIS, L. M. and PAWAN, G. L. S. (1968) Aspects of fat metabolism in anorexia nervosa. *Metabolism*, **17**, 1109–1118

CRISP, A. H. and STONEHILL, E. (1967) Hypercarotenaemia as a symptom of weight phobia. *Postgrad. Med. J.*, **43**, 721–725

CURRAN-CELENTANO, J., ERDMAN, J. W., NELSON, R. A. and GRATER, S. J. E. (1985) Alterations in vitamin A and thyroid hormone status in anorexia nervosa and associated disorders. *Am. J. Clin. Nutr.*, **42**, 1183–1191

DALLY, P. J. (1959) Carotenaemia occurring in a case of anorexia nervosa. *Br. Med. J.*, ii, 1333

FABRY, P. and TEPPERMAN, J. (1970) Meal frequency—a possible factor in human pathology. *Am. J. Clin. Nutr.*, **23**, 1059–1068

GREENE, C. H. and BLACKFORD, L. M. (1926) Carotinemia. *Med. Clin. North Am.*, **10**, 733–744

HALMI, K. and FRY, M. (1974) Serum lipids in anorexia nervosa. *Biol. Psychiatry*, **8**, 159–167

HALMI, K. A. and FALK, J. A. (1981) Common physiological changes in anorexia nervosa. *Int. J. Eating Disorders*, **1**, 16–27

HURD, H. P., PALUMBO, P. J. and GHARIB, H. (1977) Hypothalamic–endocrine dysfunction in anorexia nervosa. *Mayo Clin. Proc.*, **52**, 711–716

KANIS, J. A., BROWN, P., FITZPATRICK, K., HIBBERT, D. J., HORN, D. B., NAIRN, I. M. *et al.* (1974) Anorexia nervosa: a clinical, psychiatric and laboratory study. *Q. J. Med.*, **67**, 321–328

KEMMAN, E., PASQUALE, S. A. and SKAF, R. (1983) Amenorrhea associated with carotenemia. *J. Am. Med. Assoc.*, **249**, 926–929

KLINEFELTER, H. F. (1965) Hypercholesterolemia in anorexia nervosa. *J. Clin. Endocrinol. Metab.*, **25**, 1520–1521

LEVIN, O. L. and SILVERS, S. H. (1931) Carotinemia resulting from restricted diet as observed in dermatologic practice. *J. Am. Med. Assoc.*, **96**, 2190–2193

LUPTON, M., SIMON, L., BARRY, V. and KLAWANS, H. L. (1976) Biological aspects of anorexia nervosa. *Life Sci.*, **18**, 1341–1348

MATTINGLY, D. and BHANJI, S. (1982) The diagnosis of anorexia nervosa. *J. R. Coll. Physicians Lond.*, **16**, 191–194

MILNER, M. R., MCANARNEY, E. R. and KLISH, W. J. (1985) Metabolic abnormalities in adolescent patients with anorexia nervosa. *J. Adolesc. Health Care*, **6**, 193–195

MORDASINI, R., KLOSE, G. and GRETEN, H. (1978) Secondary type II hyperlipoproteinemia in patients with anorexia nervosa. *Metabolism*, **27**, 71–79

NESTEL, P. J. (1974) Cholesterol metabolism in anorexia nervosa and hypercholesterolemia. *J. Clin. Endocrinol. Metab.*, **38**, 325–328

POPS, M. A. and SCHWABE, A. D. (1968) Hypercarotenemia in anorexia nervosa. *J. Am. Med. Assoc.*, **205**, 533–534

ROBBOY, M. S., SATO, A. S. and SCHWABE, A. D. (1974) The hypercarotenemia in anorexia nervosa: a comparison of vitamin A and carotene levels in various forms of menstrual dysfunction and cachexia. *Am. J. Clin. Nutr.*, **27**, 362–367

SCHWABE, A. D., LIPPE, B. M., CHANG, R. J., POPS, M. A. and YAGER, J. (1981) Anorexia nervosa. *Ann. Intern. Med.*, **94**, 371–381

SHARMAN, I. M. (1985) Hypercarotenaemia. *Br. Med. J.*, **290**, 95–96

SILVERMAN, J. A. (1974) Anorexia nervosa: clinical observations in a successful treatment plan. *J. Pediatr.*, **84**, 68–73

WARREN, M. P. and VANDE WIELE, R. L. (1973) Clinical and metabolic features of anorexia nervosa. *Am. J. Obstet. Gynecol.*, **117**, 435–449

Chapter 13

Nutritional disorders

Malnutrition is not only the major feature of anorexia nervosa, but in this disorder has particular characteristics. In involuntary starvation, such as occurs under famine conditions, the major feature is deprivation of protein, often accompanied by deficiency of essential nutrients such as vitamins. By contrast, in anorexia nervosa protein intake is usually adequate and vitamin deficiency is rare. Serum protein levels are seldom below normal, and the plasma aminogram similarly has a normal appearance, quite unlike that seen in kwashiorkor (Russell, 1969). The anorectic carefully avoids carbohydrate foods, and prefers instead cheese, salads and fruit. Some will eat a little meat, fish or poultry, but it is our impression that the incidence of vegetarianism among anorectics is increasing; this, however, may merely be a reflection of current fashion among the young. The extreme vegan is often aware of the risks she runs and will request or purchase vitamin supplements.

The long-standing clinical opinion that anorectics have a high knowledge of dietary matters was confirmed in an Australian sample studied by Beumont *et al.* (1981) who found that most anorectics scored higher than matched controls on a test of nutritional knowledge. They were particularly knowledgeable about food calorie content, dieting, cooking methods and roughage, but tended to score less well on questions related to public health issues. We made slight modifications to the questionnaire, to allow for national differences in terminology, and administered it to 25 consecutive cases. Only six subjects did well and we were not able to confirm that dieters performed better than vomiters and purgers.

General effects of starvation

The most striking effect of the nutritional disturbance in anorexia nervosa is the loss of body substance. The lost tissue has been shown to consist largely of solid matter, particularly fat (Ljunggren, Ikkos and Luft, 1961; Russell, 1969; Fohlin, 1977). Some have shown that a further general consequence is retarded growth and development. Crisp (1969) found no overall difference in height between anorectics and neurotics matched for age, sex and social class, but the anorectics had narrower shoulders. Narrow hips were seen only in those aged under 18 years. The differences were attributed to oestrogen deficiency. Lacey *et al.* (1979) found delayed radiological bone age in anorexia nervosa, and suggested that bone development ceases when the fall in weight is sufficient to stop menstruation.

Toms and Crisp (1972) described a male anorectic who began to lose weight when

12 years old, at which time his height was on the fiftieth percentile for his age and he was slightly overweight. When admitted for treatment 3 years later his appearance was that of a 10 or 11 year old, and both his weight and height were below the third percentile. Not only did his weight increase in response to treatment, but growth recommenced and he developed evidence of puberty. Three more cases of anorexia nervosa presenting with retarded growth were reported by Root and Powers (1983). In all three it took over 3 years before the true diagnosis was recognized. Pugliese *et al.* (1983) described 14 children who at the age of 12 years or less began to diet because of a fear of obesity and who showed a deceleration in linear growth. Although the patients had much in common with those suffering from anorexia nervosa, and indeed would have been diagnosed as such by some, the authors regarded them as having a different disorder.

Nussbaum *et al.* (1985) investigated the heights of 85 cases of anorexia nervosa and found that over three-quarters were below the fiftieth height percentile for their age, and that anorectics were significantly shorter than their parents. As most of the patients developed anorexia after the menarche, it was suggested that malnutrition alone could not be held responsible. The authors considered the possibilities that short stature predisposed towards anorexia as it would make even a modest tendency toward obesity more noticeable, or alternatively a hypothalamic lesion was responsible for both retarded growth and anorexia nervosa. In contrast, Nielsen (1985) found no evidence of disturbed growth before the onset of anorexia nervosa, and Pfeiffer, Lucas and Ilstrup (1986) demonstrated that, in the majority of their 71 anorectics, height continued to increase at the expected rate. In those patients who did have retarded growth, this tended to increase after weight had been gained.

We were unable to demonstrate any significant effect of this disease on growth in our patients. When they presented to us, one-half were above the fiftieth percentile for height, and the other half were below it. There were no statistically significant differences between the former and the latter with regard to either the mean age of onset of the loss of weight, or the mean age at which patients presented to us.

Water-soluble vitamins

Dally and Gomez (1979) have stated that if vitamin deficiency is present the diagnosis of anorexia nervosa may have to be reconsidered. Nevertheless, isolated cases have been recorded.

Vitamin B complex

Palmer (1939) reported a 22-year-old female with a 3-year history of dieting and vomiting before complaining of tinnitus and becoming confused, restless and incontinent. On examination she was emaciated, her skin was dry and scaly, and her tongue red and glazed. There was a tachycardia, a low-grade evening pyrexia, and signs of flaccid paralysis and sensory disturbance in both legs. Beri-beri was diagnosed, and the patient responded to thiamine.

Smitt (1946) described a 41-year-old woman with a 4-year history of depression, anorexia, vomiting, weight loss and amenorrhoea. For some 2 months, she had been too weak to leave her bed and had developed marked oedema of the legs. Neurological examination revealed a depressed and apathetic mental state, general muscle weakness, reduced tendon reflexes at the knees, and impaired sensation in the legs. A chest radiograph showed a right pleural effusion. In spite of rest, fluid restriction, and a nourishing diet, there was no change in her condition. After 3 weeks thiamine was prescribed, and was followed by a dramatic improvement. About 2 weeks later, the patient developed dough-like skin over the nose and cheeks, and complained of a generalized burning sensation. She was thought to have early pellagra and was treated accordingly with success. However, on leaving hospital she was still anorectic and her gait was unsteady.

In 1982 the first report appeared of an anorectic who developed Wernicke's encephalopathy (Handler and Perkin, 1982). Unfortunately, thiamine levels could not be usefully investigated as the patient had been on a normal diet for some 6 months before she sought attention for her neurological symptoms. The authors stressed that Wernicke's encephalopathy should be suspected in any chronic anorectic with nystagmus and ataxia.

It would appear that deficiencies of nicotinic acid are just as rare as those of thiamine. Magendantz and Proger (1940) reported that they had seen an emaciated young anorectic with early signs of typical pellagra and Smitt (1946) mentioned three cases. Only one of the patients in the large series recorded by Berkman (1930) was described as pellagrous, but no details were given. Of the two anorectics discussed by Clow (1932), one had been ill for 10 years, and every other year would develop signs of pellagra such as a red scaling eruption on the back of both hands and forearms and on the front of the neck, a beefy red sore tongue, and diarrhoea. In view of her diet, which was claimed to consist of only 100 calories each day and virtually no vitamins it is likely that she also suffered from lack of other essential nutrients. Martin (1955) reported two fatal cases of anorexia nervosa. At autopsy, brain changes similar to those in pellagra were found. More recently, Rapaport (1985) described a 20-year-old female patient who developed a pruritic photosensitivity rash over the back of her hands and forearms. The serum zinc level was normal, but the skin biopsy appearance was compatible with pellagra and the urinary excretion of nicotinic acid metabolites was low. The rash disappeared, apart from some persisting pigmentation, when she was treated with oral nicotinic acid.

Vitamin C

Most anorectics will happily eat fruit, and so vitamin C deficiency is also rare. Birley (1933) made reference to two anorectics who had scurvy, and Ryle (1936) described another case with widespread purpura who died. Magenantz and Proger (1940) reported a 28-year-old woman with an 8-year history of anorexia associated with vomiting. For 2 years the vomitus had contained blood. There were no skin lesions, but Hess's test was positive and gastroscopy revealed multiple pin-point haemorrhages. George, Zabow and Beumont (1975) described scurvy and an iron deficiency anaemia in an anorectic who decided to exclude all fruits and vegetables from her diet. After 6 months she developed swollen ankles, stiff joints with painful swelling of the left knee, extensive bruising, and swollen gums which bled readily. An ascorbic acid excretion test was abnormal, confirming vitamin C deficiency. We have seen one emaciated young woman with widespread perifollicular purpura which responded to ascorbic acid.

Vitamin B_{12} and folic acid

According to Silverman (1974), lack of vitamin B_{12} or folic acid never occurs in anorexia nervosa, but Mant and Faragher (1972) found low serum folate levels in three out of seven cases; however, none showed macrocytosis. Serum B_{12} and folate concentrations were measured in 16 of our more recent patients. With the exception of one instance of a moderately reduced folate level of 2.3 µg/l all the values fell within the appropriate normal ranges. The mean red cell volume was measured in 30 of our drug-free patients. This was slightly elevated in only four, the highest value being 98.0 fl.

Fat-soluble vitamins

Vitamin A

Silverman (1974) found low serum retinol (vitamin A) levels in 14 (67%) of his anorectics, but none of the 10 who had slit-lamp examinations showed any abnormality. Abraham, Banks and Beumont (1980) also failed to find any ophthalmological signs of vitamin A deficiency, although most of their patients had vitamin A intakes below the recommended level. Other work suggests that serum retinol concentrations are normal or even elevated in this disease (Robboy, Sato and Schwabe, 1974; Casper et al., 1980; Langan and Farrell, 1985). This latter finding is not altogether surprising when one considers the raised levels of serum β-carotene in many patients. This substance is a precursor of vitamin A and has been discussed in more detail in the previous chapter.

Vitamin D

Osteoporosis has occasionally been reported in patients with anorexia nervosa, but there is no convincing evidence to suggest that vitamin D deficiency contributes to the thinning of the bones (Riggotti et al., 1984; Szmukler et al., 1985; Kaplan et al., 1986; Treasure, Fogelman and Russell, 1986). Nevertheless, Fonseca et al. (1985) found that the mean serum 25-hydroxyvitamin D levels in 16 anorectics were lower than in their control subjects, and Crosby et al. (1985) reported low vitamin D intakes in most of their patients. Only one of our cases had definite biochemical evidence of osteomalacia. The serum calcium, phosphate and alkaline phosphatase levels returned rapidly to normal following the administration of calciferol.

Vitamin E

We know of no reports of vitamin E (tocopherol) deficiency in this disorder. Langan and Farrell (1985) found no shortage of total tocopherol, nor of the major and most active isomer, α-tocopherol, in their series. Plasma levels of β- and γ-tocopherols, which are found only in food and not synthesized by the body, were however somewhat reduced.

Vitamin K

Purpura due to a deficiency of vitamin K has been described by Aggeler, Lucia and Fishbow (1942) in a 32-year-old patient with a long history of anorexia, vomiting and diarrhoea. During various times in her illness she had been troubled by bleeding gums and ecchymoses, and at one stage bled into her elbow joints. Repeated large doses of ascorbic acid had been without effect. On presentation, there were numerous ecchymoses, and the gums were spongy and bleeding. Investigations revealed a prolonged clotting time. The serum ascorbic acid level was low, but capillary fragility was normal. The patient responded well to the administration of synthetic vitamin K. The rarity of vitamin K lack in anorexia nervosa is illustrated by the normal prothrombin times in all 40 cases studied by Halmi and Falk (1981).

Fatty acids

Essential fatty acids are the precursors of prostaglandins, and are also important components of cell membranes. Clinical manifestations of deficiency include dry scaly skin, prolonged wound healing, and thrombocytopenia. All of these are seen from time to time in anorectic patients, but may have other causes. Langan and Farrell (1985) investigated essential fatty acid status in 17 anorectics. Analysis of the plasma phospholipid fraction revealed abnormally low levels of linoleate and the absence of linolenate. The ratio of linoleate to arachidonate was reduced, providing evidence of a decreased intake of essential fatty acids.

Amino acids

Severe protein deficiency is thought to be rare in anorexia nervosa, despite the obvious wasting of the skeletal muscles in severe cases. The plasma aminogram does not reveal any deficiency of essential amino acids in this disorder (Russell, 1969). We know of only one report of kwashiorkor resulting from anorexia nervosa (Esca *et al.*, 1979). They described a 26-year-old white teacher who existed on a diet of alcohol and pickled cucumbers for 4 months, during which time she lost 20 kg in weight and developed acrodermatitis enteropathica. On examination she also had pallor, loss of hair pigment, and an enlarged liver. She was found to be hypoproteinaemic, hypocalcaemic, hypokalaemic, and to have abnormal liver function tests as well as a low serum zinc level. Replacement therapy with oral zinc and intravenous human albumin resulted in a rapid and lasting remission of her skin and biochemical abnormalities.

Trace elements

Zinc

There have been relatively few studies of trace elements in anorexia nervosa. Casper *et al.* (1980) evaluated zinc, copper and iron levels in 30 anorectics and 33 healthy controls. Although the hair contained normal amounts of zinc, the mean serum and urinary zinc concentrations were significantly lower in the anorectics. The plasma zinc level did not correlate with the duration or extent of weight loss, nor with the plasma concentrations of carotene, retinol or retinol binding protein; nor was there any correlation between plasma zinc concentrations and taste threshold in the 20 anorectics tested for hypogeusia. Ainley *et al.* (1986) have pointed out that urine, plasma and hair zinc levels do not reflect tissue zinc status, and that a more reliable method is to estimate the neutrophil zinc concentration. Using this technique they found that only three out of 14 anorectics were zinc deficient. However, there are some reports of anorectics with acrodermatitis enteropathica which responded to zinc supplements (Thomsen, 1978; Esca et al., 1979).

We estimated the serum zinc concentrations in 14 of our patients. Eight had concentrations below the normal range, the lowest level being 5.7 µmol/l. Only one, who had a serum zinc concentration of 7.0 µmol/l, complained of hypogeusia. Oral zinc supplements were given to three patients, but we were unable to demonstrate any convincing effect on appetite or weight gain.

Copper

Hoes (1977) reported that plasma copper concentrations were low in five out of six cases of anorexia nervosa, and stated that the patients responded well to oral copper sulphate given for 5 weeks. Casper et al. (1980) also found that plasma copper levels were low, but the hair copper content was normal and there was no reduction in serum ceruloplasmin. Copper depletion was not sufficient to affect adversely haemoglobin synthesis. After treatment consisting of a diet including mineral and vitamin supplements, psychotherapy and behaviour therapy, the serum copper and ceruloplasmin levels increased.

Summary

Nutritional deficiency diseases are surprisingly rare in anorexia nervosa, despite the grossly emaciated state of some of the patients. Investigation for such disorders may prove rewarding if unexpected symptoms or signs are encountered, particularly in those on bizarre diets. There is no convincing evidence at present to suggest that zinc or copper deficiency plays a role in the aetiology of this disorder.

References

ABRAHAM, S. F., BANKS, C. N. and BEUMONT, P. J. V. (1980) Eye signs in patients with anorexia nervosa. *Aust. J. Ophthalmol.*, **8**, 55–57

AGGELER, P. M., LUCIA, S. P. and FISHBOW, H. M. (1942) Purpura due to vitamin K deficiency in anorexia nervosa. *J. Dig. Dis.*, **9**, 227–229

AINLEY, C. E., CASON, J., CARLSSON, L., THOMPSON, R. P. H., SLAVIN, B. M. and NORTON, K. R. W. (1986) Zinc state in anorexia nervosa. *Br. Med. J.*, **293**, 992–993

BERKMAN, J. M. (1930) Anorexia nervosa, anorexia, inanation, and low basal metabolic rate. *Am. J. Med. Sci.*, **180**, 411–424

BEUMONT, P. J. V., CHAMBERS, T. L., ROUSE, L. and ABRAHAM, S. F. (1981) The diet composition and nutritional knowledge of patients with anorexia nervosa. *J. Hum. Nutr.*, **35**, 263–273

BIRLEY, J. L. (1933) Anorexia nervosa. *St Thomas's Hospital Gazette*, **34**, 204–208

CASPER, R. C., KIRSCHNER, B., SANDSTEAD, H. H., JACOB, R. A. and DAVIS, J. M. (1980) An evaluation of trace metals, vitamins, and taste function in anorexia nervosa. *Am. J. Clin. Nutr.*, **33**, 1801–1808

CLOW, F. E. (1932) Anorexia nervosa. *N. Eng. J. Med.*, **207**, 613–617

CRISP, A. H. (1969) Some skeletal measurements in patients with primary anorexia nervosa. *J. Psychosom. Res.*, **13**, 125–142

CROSBY, L. O., KAPLAN, F. S., PERTSCHUK, M. J. and MULLEN, J. L. (1985) The effects of anorexia nervosa on bone morphometry in young women. *Clin. Orthop.*, **201**, 271–277

DALLY, P. and GOMEZ, J. (1979) *Anorexia nervosa*. London: William Heinemann Medical Books Ltd

ESCA, S. A., BRENNER, W., MACH, K. and GSCHNAIT, F. (1979) Kwashiorkor-like zinc deficiency syndrome in anorexia nervosa. *Acta Derm. Venereol.*, **59**, 361–364

FOHLIN, L. (1977) Body composition, cardiovascular and renal function in adolescent patients with anorexia nervosa. *Acta Paediatr. Scand.*, suppl. 268

FONSECA, V., HOULDER, S., THOMAS, M., D'SOUZA, V., WAKELING, A. and DANDONA, P. (1985) Osteopenia in women with anorexia nervosa. *N. Eng. J. Med.*, **313**, 326

GEORGE, G. C. W., ZABOW, T. and BEUMONT, P. J. V. (1975) Scurvy in anorexia nervosa. *S. Afr. Med. J.*, **49**, 1420

HALMI, K. A. and FALK, J. A. (1981) Common physiological changes in anorexia nervosa. *Int. J. Eating Disorders*, **1**, 16–27

HANDLER, C. E. and PERKIN, G. D. (1982) Anorexia nervosa and Wernicke's encephalopathy: an underdiagnosed association. *Lancet*, ii, 771–772

HOES, M. A. J. A. M. (1977) Copper, pimozide treatment for anorexia nervosa. *Proceedings of the VIth World Congress of Psychiatry*, p. 156

KAPLAN, F. S., PERTSCHUK, M., FALLON, M. and HADDAD, J. (1986) Osteoporosis and hip fracture in a young woman with anorexia nervosa. *Clin. Orthop.*, **212**, 250–254

LACEY, J. H., CRISP, A. H., HART, G. and KIRKWOOD, B. A. (1979) Weight and skeletal maturation—a study of radiological and chronological age in an anorexia nervosa population. *Postgrad. Med. J.*, **55**, 381–385

LANGAN, S. M. and FARRELL, P. M. (1985) Vitamin E, vitamin A and essential fatty acid status of patients hospitalized for anorexia nervosa. *Am. J. Clin. Nutr.*, **41**, 1054–1060

LJUNGGREN, H., IKKOS, D. and LUFT, R. (1961) Basal metabolism in women with obesity and anorexia nervosa. *Br. J. Nutr.*, **15**, 21–34

MAGENDANTZ, H. and PROGER, S. (1940) Anorexia nervosa or hypopituitarism. *J. Am. Med. Assoc.*, **114**, 1973–1983

MANT, M. J. and FARAGHER, B. S. (1972) The haematology of anorexia nervosa. *Br. J. Haematol.*, **23**, 737–749

MARTIN, F. (1955) Pathologie des aspects neurologiques et psychiatriques dans quelque manifestations carentielles avec troubles digestifs et neuro-endocriniens. II Etudes des alterations du systeme nerveux central dans deux cas d'anorexie survenue chez la jeune fille (dite anorexie mentale). *Helv. Med. Acta.*, **22**, 522–529

NIELSEN, S. (1985) Evaluation of growth in anorexia nervosa from serial measurements. *J. Psychiatr. Res.*, **19**, 227–230

NUSSBAUM, M., BAIRD, D., SONNENBLICK, M., COWAN, K. and SHENKER, I. R. (1985) Short stature in anorexia nervosa patients. *J. Adolesc. Health Care*, **6**, 453–455

PALMER, H. A. (1939) Beriberi complicating anorexia nervosa. *Lancet*, i, 269

PFEIFFER, R. J., LUCAS, A. R. and ILSTRUP, D. M. (1986) Effect of anorexia nervosa on linear growth. *Clin. Pediatr.*, **25**, 7–12

PUGLIESE, M. T., LIFSHITZ, F., GRAD, G., FORT, P. and MARKS-KATZ, M. (1983) Fear of obesity: a cause of short stature and delayed puberty. *N. Engl. J. Med.*, **309**, 513–518

RAPAPORT, M. J. (1985) Pellagra in a patient with anorexia nervosa. *Arch Dermatol.*, **121**, 255–257

RIGOTTI, N. A., NUSSBAUM, S. R., HERZOG, D. B. and NEER, R. M. (1984) Osteoporosis in women with anorexia nervosa. *N. Engl. J. Med.*, **311**, 1601–1606

ROBBOY, M. S., SATO, A. S. and SCHWABE, A. D. (1974) The hypercarotenemia in anorexia nervosa: a comparison of vitamin A and carotene levels in various forms of menstrual dysfunction and cachexia. *Am. J. Clin. Nutr.*, **27**, 362–367

ROOT, A. W. and POWERS, P. S. (1983) Anorexia nervosa presenting as growth retardation in adolescents. *J. Adolesc. Health Care*, **4**, 25–30

RUSSELL, G. F. M. (1969) Metabolic, endocrine and psychiatric aspects of anorexia nervosa. *Scientific Basis of Medicine Annual Review*, **16**, 236–255

RYLE, J. A. (1936) Anorexia nervosa. *Lancet*, ii, 893–899

SILVERMAN, J. A. (1974) Anorexia nervosa: clinical observations in a successful treatment plan. *J. Pediatr.*, **84**, 68–73

SMITT, J. W. (1946) Case of anorexia nervosa complicated by beriberi. *Acta Psychiatr. Neurol.*, **21**, 887–900

SZMUKLER, G. I., BROWN, S. W., PARSONS, V. and DARBY, A. (1985) Premature loss of bone in chronic anorexia nervosa. *Br. Med. J.*, **290**, 26–27

THOMSEN, K. (1978) Zinc, liver cirrhosis and anorexia nervosa. *Acta Derm. Venereol.*, **58**, 283

TOMS, D. A. and CRISP, A. H. (1972) Weight phobia in an adolescent male with stunted development. *J. Psychosom. Res.*, **16**, 289–295

TREASURE, J., FOGELMAN, I. and RUSSELL, G. F. M. (1986) Osteopaenia of the lumbar spine and femoral neck in anorexia nervosa. *Scott. Med. J.*, **31**, 206–207

Chapter 14

Psychiatric management

Although this book is concerned primarily with the medical aspects of anorexia nervosa, we hope that this brief account of the principles and practice of psychiatric treatment will not be regarded as out of place. It appears that anorectics are referred equally to physicians and psychiatrists (Bhanji, 1979), and so it is likely that patients seen in the general hospital may well have received psychiatric care in the past or are being treated jointly by psychiatric and medical teams. The following account is of necessity a superficial one; the reader interested in more information should consult the standard psychiatric texts, or those on anorexia nervosa which devote substantial space to the psychiatric and psychological aspects of the disorder. According to their approach to the aetiology and management of mental disturbance, psychiatrists can be characterized as belonging to one of three types: organic, psychodynamic, or behavioural.

The approach of the organic psychiatrist

The organic psychiatrist regards mental illness as basically no different from physical disease. Psychotic illness, for example, is seen as deriving from inherited or acquired disturbances in brain neurotransmission. Although there is evidence that this may apply to schizophrenia and manic depressive psychosis, it is far from conclusive. Nevertheless, treatment derived from this view does appear to be effective. Neurotic disorders are regarded as no more than understandable reactions to a stressful situation by a person with a vulnerable personality, and as therefore perhaps better dealt with by the lay psychotherapist, social worker, or clinical psychologist rather than by a doctor. With regard to anorexia nervosa attitudes vary. Some organically-orientated psychiatrists see their role as correcting, by medical means, a hypothalamic disorder; the majority, however, base their treatment on empirical evidence that it produces a gain in weight.

The treatments employed consist mainly of drugs and methods such as electroconvulsive therapy (ECT), or more rarely modified insulin therapy and psychosurgery. Unless there is evidence of severe depression ECT should not, as has happened in the past, be given as a matter of course. Similarly, most people believe that the management of anorexia nervosa has now advanced sufficiently to render psychosurgery obsolete. The use of insulin and other forms of drug therapy are discussed in Chapters 15 and 16.

The psychodynamic approach

The psychodynamic psychiatrists stand in marked contrast to their organically-orientated colleagues in that they prefer to emphasize the importance of psychological and social factors in determining abnormal mental phenomena. They view their remit as broader than that of the organic psychiatrist, being pleased to regard neurosis as an illness which they can treat appropriately.

The basis of psychodynamic theory and practice is that neurotic and psychotic symptoms stem from unconscious mental conflict. In its simplest form, derived from the teachings of Freud, this relates to an early traumatic event, usually of a sexual nature. As any recollection of the incident would provoke intolerable anxiety, the memory of what happened is kept securely away from consciousness. This process is known as repression, and is sometimes assisted by the generation of a false memory to replace the true one. If in later life an event which bears resemblance to the original occurs, repression may partially fail. The patient may then become apparently unaccountably anxious, or may develop other symptoms. The latter depend on which defence mechanisms are employed. The function of these defence mechanisms is to allow the release of emotional tension, but in such a way that the cause remains concealed. Remarks on a girl's developing sexual attractiveness made by male members of the family could threaten the sanctity of repressed memories of an early incestuous episode. Displacement could then serve to transform sexual anxiety into a fear of food or of fatness and lead to anorexia nervosa. The preoccupation with the calorific content of foods in this disorder may represent the sublimation of sexual feelings, and the desire to remain anchored in the security of childhood may be due to regression.

Symbolization is another important defence mechanism and has been invoked to explain how particular physical symptoms or signs arise from emotional stress. Many early psychosomatic theories were developed by those with a background in psychoanalysis. Hence the emphasis placed on such symbolic aspects of anorexia nervosa as eating representing impregnation, and fatness pregnancy. There are now many branches of the psychodynamic movement. By no means all agree over the primacy of sexual matters, and many concentrate on the way more general childhood events and relationships can affect behaviour in later life.

Interpretive psychotherapy

The mainstay of psychodynamic treatment is interpretive psychotherapy. Here the aim is to expose, explore and explain the relevant unconscious problem. In doing so some use the traditional Freudian techniques of free association and dream analysis, but others have derived less rigorous and time-consuming forms of psychotherapy. From a practical point of view the physician should be aware of certain ground rules which may affect his management of those anorectics who are receiving psychodynamic therapy. Appointments with the therapist are generally for a fixed time and are expected to be rigidly adhered to. Contact with the patient outside these sessions is not permitted—no matter how disturbed she may become while on the medical ward. The therapist will deliberately refrain from discussing medical matters with the patient, and will expect the physician to behave similarly regarding any emotional topics. If joint discussion of the case is called for, the therapist may insist that the patient and family be present.

Supportive psychotherapy

Although interpretive psychotherapy has its adherents, mainly from outside the medical profession, the general view is that its value in anorexia nervosa is limited, particularly if it consists of traditional psychoanalysis. Hence many psychotherapists prefer supportive psychotherapy where the emphasis is on the present and the future rather than the past, and where practical as well as emotional issues can be discussed. A fact-finding approach has been favoured as it helps the anorectic recognize that she has emotions and experiences of her own. So-called insight imposed from without serves only to reinforce her anger at having always to acquiesce. The therapist is usually amenable to seeing the patient at short notice if the situation is urgent. Psychological and medical aspects are not necessarily regarded as separate issues, and many psychiatrists practising this form of therapy are prepared to deal with both.

Supportive psychotherapy on its own is probably of greatest value in those anorectics who seek help early, and where the precipitating event is clear and can be dealt with. However, even in the chronic cases with marked loss of weight, it can provide a valuable adjunct to other therapeutic measures.

The behavioural approach

The behavioural approach dismisses unconscious conflict as the cause of mental illness and requires that symptoms are treated in their own right and not as the superficial manifestations of something else. The existence of an unconscious region of the mind is not disputed, but its significance is. Put succinctly, the behaviourist believes that people are as they are because they have learned to be that way.

This learning process takes two basic forms, the first being by classical, or Pavlovian, conditioning. Thus, if meals happen to coincide with an unpleasant event, such as an episode of nausea or a family argument, an aversion to food may develop and persist long after the coincident event has ceased to occur. The other form of learning depends on operant conditioning. Here the important factor is not the concurrence of stimuli, but the effect of a particular response. If the response results in pleasurable events it is more likely to be repeated than if something unpleasant happens. An adolescent girl may one day be off her food; her mother reacts with solicitous attention, and so refusing food comes to have its rewards. If drastic dieting ensues and the concern aroused serves to re-unite a previously divided family, there is further inducement to continue. The disappearance of an unpleasant consequence is just as potent a reinforcer as the arrival of a pleasing one. The girl who is no longer teased because she is overweight may be sorely tempted to continue to diet even though her weight is now normal.

In contrast to the psychodynamic therapists, who have often been criticized for their complacency over theories which many see as lacking any scientific foundation, the behaviourists have been attacked for their over-scientific mechanistic attitude toward the complexities of human life. Whatever the rights and wrongs of this debate, there is much evidence that for the relief of any given symptom behaviour therapy compares favourably with psychodynamic therapy. Hence the preference for behaviour therapy among those psychiatrists who treat anorectics.

Systematic desensitization

Systematic desensitization involves treating anorexia nervosa as a phobia of eating, and utilizes techniques used to allay other irrational fears. The patient is gradually exposed to the aversive stimulus, being helped to feel relaxed and calm at each stage. Eventually a state of panic is replaced by one of equanimity. Exposure to the stimulus may be in the real situation or one which resembles it, or may take place in the patient's imagination. The psychiatrist may rely on his soothing presence to induce the necessary calmness, or may employ relaxation therapy or a short-acting tranquillizer.

Systematic desensitization is most effective when the phobia is for a specific object or situation. Because of this its effectiveness in anorexia nervosa has been limited, and most psychiatrists who favour behaviour therapy use operant conditioning as this is more appropriate to the alteration of complex behaviour patterns.

Operant conditioning

Without realizing it, many physicians have been using operant conditioning for well over a century. The anorectic is put to bed and told she will not be allowed up or to go home until her weight is satisfactory. Intermediate rewards before the final one of discharge from hospital include warm approval from the staff. The behaviour therapist, however, prefers a more formalized regimen set up according to certain principles. The most important of these is that operant conditioning should be carried out only with the full knowledge and consent of the patient and her family. The second most important point to be borne in mind is that rewarding appropriate behaviour is more effective than punishing undesirable acts; these are best ignored. The intermediate targets and the ultimate one signalling the completion of treatment should be specified in advance, as must be their rewards. Once a goal has been achieved the reward should follow as soon as possible. The targets are usually drawn up by those carrying out the treatment. The rewards are chosen by the patient, and are then given in inverse order of preference as successive targets are reached. A stipulated rate of weight gain is the commonest target, but in some programmes it is the amount of food consumed. The successful application of operant conditioning calls for constant vigilance, as patients are adept at surreptitiously disposing of food or may enhance their weight by drinking copious amounts of water or concealing weights in their clothes. Some will also obtain rewards independently; a fairly easy matter in the case of cigarettes.

In spite of its disadvantages, operant conditioning can result in rates of weight gain better than those obtained by psychotherapy alone and comparable to those achieved by medical means. Unfortunately the long-term benefits are as disappointing as with any other treatment. An early review of operant conditioning in anorexia nervosa was provided by Bhanji (1975). A more recent discussion is presented by Garfinkel and Garner (1982). One of the main criticisms of behaviour therapy, particularly operant conditioning, is that it ignores the personal factors which led to the anorexia nervosa. Furthermore, by taking control over the patient the therapist runs the risk of perpetuating the loss of individuality and sense of ineffectiveness which is so often a feature of this disorder.

Behaviour therapy produces rapid weight gain but ignores the wider issues. Psychodynamic therapy on the other hand is directed at what many psychiatrists regard as the cause, but takes much longer to carry out. Nowadays the two approaches are often combined. In many instances psychotherapy is substituted for behaviour therapy once the patient has regained weight; indeed the prospect of psychotherapy may be the final incentive in a behavioural programme. An alternative is to combine the two right from the start.

Family therapy

Since the first report by Minuchin and his colleagues (Liebman, Minuchin and Baker, 1974) of the results of simultaneous behaviour therapy and family psychotherapy their approach to the psychiatric management of anorexia nervosa has received much support. After a period of observation, during which the staff join the patient for lunch, it is stipulated that the anorectic will be allowed out of bed only if her weight has increased by half a pound during the previous day. A week or so later the family, the paediatrician, and the psychiatrist have another lunch with the patient. At the end of this meal, a target weight for discharge home is agreed. After the patient has left the hospital the family carry on with a behavioural regimen and are supported by the therapist.

Summary

There is a variety of psychiatric techniques available for the treatment of anorexia nervosa. Regrettably, in the past these were often selected according to the psychiatrist's orientation rather than on the basis of proven effectiveness. In recent years there has been a refreshing tendency toward greater open-mindedness on the part of the psychiatrist and it is now not uncommon to use two or more treatment methods either concurrently or in sequence. In general terms, regimens relying heavily on behaviour therapy produce the best short-term results, and those in which family therapy plays the major role are thought to be the most effective in the long-term.

References

BHANJI, S. (1975) Operant conditioning in anorexia nervosa. In *Current Psychiatric Therapies, Vol. 15*, edited by J. Masserman, pp. 59–64. New York: Grune and Stratton

BHANJI, S. (1979) Anorexia nervosa: physicians' and psychiatrists' opinions and practice. *J. Psychosom. Res.*, **23**, 7–11

GARFINKEL, P. E. and GARNER, D. M. (1982) *Anorexia nervosa: a Multidimensional Perspective*. New York: Brunner/Mazel

LIEBMAN, R., MINUCHIN, S. and BAKER, L. (1974) An integrated treatment program for anorexia nervosa. *Am. J. Psychiatry*, **131**, 432–436

Chapter 15

Medical management

The early physicians treating this disorder thought little of the drugs available to them and relied upon removing the patient from the influence of family and friends, bed rest and warmth, and exhortations to eat a nourishing diet. Many still base their general management on this. Tube feeding was among the first specific measures, but has now fallen out of favour. The decline in the use of tube feeding coincided with a renewed interest in medication. Writing a decade ago Bemis (1978) mentioned the extraordinary variety of somatic remedies which had been advocated at various times during the previous half century. These included thyroid extract, implanted calves' pituitary, vitamins, insulin, ACTH, corticosteroids, testosterone, anabolic agents, L-dopa, and antipsychotic (neuroleptic) drugs.

Tube feeding

A number of authors have advocated the use of tube feeding in resistive cases. In some of the patients described a duodenal tube remained in site for many weeks before the patient was willing to be fed normally. A notable exception to the view that tube feeding should be used only as a last resort was that expressed by Williams (1958) who reported on the treatment and progress of 53 female anorectics admitted to the London Hospital between 1897 and 1957. His data suggested that inpatient treatment was ineffective except in those patients who had been intubated. His recommendation that tube feeding be more freely adopted aroused much criticism and was not widely followed. A survey carried out among physicians in the UK shows that very few now use this form of treatment (Bhanji, 1979). An alternative when faced with an uncooperative, emaciated patient with severe metabolic disturbances is the use of intravenous nutrition.

Total parenteral nutrition

Finkelstein (1972) reported on two cases who, although not typical, had been diagnosed as anorexia nervosa and were in a cachectic state. A major factor in their recovery appeared to have been intravenous feeding via subclavian vein catheterization. The usefulness of intravenous nutrition in this condition was supported by a report of a patient who developed acute renal failure secondary to acute tubular necrosis and in whom an intravenous infusion of a solution of dextrose and amino acids proved life-saving (Hirschman, Rao and Chan, 1977). Maloney and Farrell (1980) described four less complicated cases in whom parenteral feeding succeeded in increasing both the patients' weights and their willingness to cooperate with psychotherapy, all other measures having failed. In contrast, Pertschuk *et al.* (1981) have drawn attention to the potential hazards of total parenteral nutrition. Of the 11 patients they described two developed peripheral weakness and numbness, followed by pneumonia. In both cases, one of whom died, the neurological complications were found to be due to hypophosphataemia. One patient suffered a pneumothorax, and another was troubled by painful joints. A transient elevation of serum transaminase levels occurred in five cases.

Pharmacotherapy

Recent reviews such as those of Johnson, Stuckey and Mitchell (1983), Crisp (1984) and Russell (1985) suggest that four main factors play a part in the decision to use any particular drug. The first is that the chosen drug has been shown to produce weight gain in other conditions. The weight-sustaining effect of insulin in the diabetic and the hunger which may result from hypoglycaemia are well recognized, but it is not clear how other drugs may cause weight gain. The neuroleptics may do so by reducing activity, producing water retention, altering carbohydrate metabolism, or blocking the actions of hypothalamic dopaminergic neurons. The antidepressants appear to induce a craving for carbohydrates, and cyproheptadine was found to increase the appetites of young asthmatics. Manic depressives on lithium may also put on weight. Finally, delta-tetrahydrocannabinol has been shown to enhance the appetites of those suffering from the late stages of cancer. However, it does not appear to be of any value in anorexia nervosa (Gross *et al.*, 1983).

The second factor is that anorexia nervosa may result from disturbances in the neurotransmitters concerned with eating. Barry and Klawans (1976) have argued that the disorder is caused by an increase in hypothalamic dopaminergic activity. Hence the dopamine antagonists, such as the neuroleptics, may be effective. If their view, that the excess dopaminergic activity results from a defective feed-back mechanism is correct, L-dopa should also be effective. An alternative theory is that anorexia nervosa results from a deficiency of hypothalamic catecholamines, especially dopamine (Mawson, 1974). Studies of the effects of both L-dopa and the dopamine agonist, bromocriptine, in anorexia nervosa have produced inconclusive findings (Johanson and Knorr, 1977; Harrower *et al.*, 1977).

The role of noradrenaline in the aetiology is uncertain, although there is some evidence that its metabolism may be abnormal in some cases and that it has different effects on feeding according to whether α- or β-receptors are involved. Redmond, Swann and Heninger (1977) administered the α-adrenergic blocker, phenoxybenzamine, to an anorectic and found that, unlike the β-adrenergic blocker, propranolol, it resulted in a gain in weight. Serotonin may act within the lateral hypothalamus to promote feelings of satiety, and the use of its antagonists is mentioned later in this chapter.

As regards other neurotransmitters, it has been suggested that in anorexia nervosa there is an excess of brain opioids. The use of the opioid antagonist, naloxone, is discussed below. Another view is that the disorder results from the hypothalamus being hypersensitive to oestrogen. If this were the case the condition might respond to progesterone (Young, 1975).

The third factor underlying the pharmacological treatment of anorexia nervosa is that it is a variant of some other disorder. Many have commented on the features that the condition shares with depressive illness, and a number of antidepressants have been used in its treatment. The association between the two states, however, has recently been questioned (Altshuler and Weiner, 1985). A substantial proportion of anorectics have abnormal EEGs; hence the use of anticonvulsants.

Finally, there is the opinion that the effects of drug therapy, albeit useful, are non-specific. Crisp (1985), for example, does not believe that chlorpromazine has any direct effect on appetite or weight: it serves merely to render the patient less frightened and less active. Similarly, Dally (1981) has stated that benzodiazepines have no effect on encouraging eating, but may be valuable in reducing anxiety over being in hospital. Those medical treatments which are the subject of current attention are now considered in more detail.

Insulin

The use of insulin in the treatment of anorexia nervosa began soon after its discovery, the earliest report we have obtained being that of Andersen (1928). Clow (1932) mentioned a patient who had been treated on a number of occasions and gained weight most rapidly when given insulin. Some, however, were not impressed. Ryle (1936) stated that insulin was of no value either in inducing hunger or in utilizing ingested carbohydrates. McCullagh and Tupper (1940) mentioned that many of their anorectics were highly sensitive to insulin, but that its beneficial effects were decidedly limited. Bond (1949) similarly noted that although hypoglycaemia developed readily this had no effect on the patient's weight. Because of the potentially serious consequences of hypoglycaemia, insulin is now rarely given to anorectics. Nevertheless we believe that it can be of considerable value in combination with neuroleptic drugs, provided that small doses are prescribed initially and the patient closely observed.

Neuroleptics

The treatment of anorexia nervosa using the neuroleptic, chlorpromazine, began shortly after its introduction some 30 years ago. In 1958 Sargant and his associates (Dally, Oppenheim and Sargant, 1958) reported that they had been using insulin for some years, but had found it to be ineffective on its own. Adding chlorpromazine in doses of up to 1000 mg daily reduced the patients' resistance toward eating and produced a greater increase in weight than insulin alone. Crisp (1965) described 21 anorectics treated with chlorpromazine, the highest dose being 600 mg each day, and found it to be a valuable adjunct to bed rest, encouragement to eat, and psychotherapy. Unfortunately, the use of chlorpromazine not infrequently resulted in side-effects, the most serious being epileptic seizures. Hence its use in anorexia nervosa fell into disrepute, even among its earlier protagonists (Dally, 1981; Crisp, 1984).

In recent years the view that anorexia nervosa stems from hyperactivity of hypothalamic dopaminergic neurons has renewed interest in the treatment of the disorder with neuroleptics such as pimozide and sulpiride which, unlike chlorpromazine, appear to be pure dopamine antagonists. Plantey (1977) reported a single case treated with 12 mg of pimozide daily. By the end of the third week the boy had gained 9 kg in weight and had lost his morbid preoccupation concerning his size. Vandereycken and Pierloot (1982) carried out a double-blind cross-over study of single daily doses of either 4 or 6 mg of pimozide and a placebo in 18 anorectics who were also receiving behaviour therapy. The patients tended to gain more weight while taking pimozide, but this effect was neither dose-related nor statistically significant. Those who did respond tended to be older and more chronic. Vandereycken (1984) carried out a similar trial of sulpiride. This drug was associated with greater daily weight increments, but as with pimozide this was not a statistically significant finding.

Antidepressants

Paykel, Mueller and De La Vergne (1973) were the first to carry out a systematic study of weight gain as a side-effect of antidepressant drugs. Their subjects were 51 female depressives who had responded to amitriptyline and were receiving maintenance therapy, placebo or no medication. Those taking amitriptyline showed gains in weight, sometimes substantial, which appeared to be dose-related and due in the main to a craving for carbohydrates. These effects were not merely due to recovery from depression, nor to hypoglycaemia or abnormal insulin tolerance. A recent investigation by Harris, Young and Hughes (1986) has compared the effects of seven antidepressant regimens on appetite, weight and preference for carbohydrates. Depressed patients were given amitriptyline, trimipramine, phenelzine, isocarboxazid, flupenthixol, trimipramine plus phenelzine, or trimipramine plus isocarboxazid. The last of these treatments resulted in the greatest increases in appetite, weight and liking for carbohydrates. Of the conventional antidepressants phenelzine had the least effect, but resulted in the second largest increase in weight when combined with trimipramine.

Monoamine oxidase inhibitors
Dally (1981) stated that there was little place for the monoamine oxidase inhibitors, but added that the depressed chronic anorectic may respond to a combination of trimipramine and tranylcypromine. Hudson *et al.* (1985) have described such a case who was eventually successfully treated with tranylcypromine and L-tryptophan. The impression that the monoamine oxidase inhibitors are usually of little value has been confirmed by an open trial of isocarboxazid (Kennedy, Piran and Garfinkel, 1985).

Monoamine reuptake inhibitors
Lacey and Crisp (1980) conducted a double-blind comparison of clomipramine and a placebo. Their patients were also being treated with bed rest, a 2600 calorie diet and individual psychotherapy. Those on clomipramine showed increased hunger, appetite and calorie intake, and became more active. They gained weight more slowly, however, but afterwards maintained their weights better than those who had received the placebo. On the other hand, a double-blind study of amitriptyline and placebo has shown that the antidepressant possessed no advantages and could cause troublesome side-effects (Biederman *et al.*, 1985). More recently, Halmi *et al.* (1986) compared the effects of amitriptyline, cyproheptadine and placebo. The investigation was double-blind and involved 72 patients treated at two hospitals. Amitriptyline proved little better than the placebo. The major influences on the outcome of treatment were the hospital at which the patient was treated, and the weight on admission.

Lithium

Kerry, Liebling and Owen (1970) reported on eight manic depressives who gained weight while receiving prophylactic lithium and suggested that this was due to an increase in solid tissue rather than to fluid retention. This was followed by other similar accounts, and an open trial of lithium carbonate in two chronic cases of anorexia nervosa who, in addition, showed some features similar to those of hypomania (Barcai, 1977). Both these patients gained weight. Gross *et al.* (1981) carried out a double-blind study in which eight patients received lithium and eight were given a placebo. In addition they all received behaviour therapy, and where necessary were tube-fed. The mean rate of weight restoration in those on the placebo was 0.19 kg/day, compared with 0.24 kg/day in those who were lithium treated. The differences in rate of weight gain were significant during the third and fourth weeks of treatment. Although these results were encouraging, it was suggested that lithium should be used only with caution and when the patients can be closely monitored. In particular, the anorectic who has cardiac complications or is hypokalaemic may be at serious risk of side-effects.

Antiserotonergic drugs

The first report to suggest that cyproheptadine may be effective in anorexia nervosa was that of Benady (1970) and described a young patient who responded to a combination of cyproheptadine 12 mg daily and weekly psychotherapy, having failed to benefit from a variety of medical and psychiatric treatments. Subsequent double-blind trials have, however, shown that this drug has few, if any, advantages over placebo (Vigersky and Loriaux, 1977; Goldberg *et al.*, 1979; Halmi *et al.*, 1986). Dolecek and Janstova (1985) have reported that another antiserotonergic agent, pizotifen, may cause weight gain, but this has not yet been confirmed.

Anticonvulsants

Green and Rau (1974) reported that four anorectics, all of whom had abnormal EEGs and periodically binged, responded well to phenytoin 100 mg thrice daily. Subsequent work has suggested that the main role of this drug may be in controlling compulsive overeating, rather than as a possible remedy for any underlying anorexia nervosa (Wermuth *et al.*, 1977; Rau, Struve and Green, 1979). Frequent binging was a prominent symptom in an anorectic who was described as responding well to a combination of carbamazepine and lithium (Hudson *et al.*, 1985).

Metoclopramide

Metoclopramide has three effects of possible relevance to anorexia nervosa. First, it increases stomach emptying by increasing gastric peristalsis, relaxing the pylorus and duodenum, and increasing tonus in the lower end of the oesophagus. Second, it acts on the medullary vomiting centre to produce an antiemetic effect. Finally, it may block dopaminergic nervous transmission within the hypothalamus. Saleh and Lebwohl (1980) confirmed that food tends to accumulate in the stomach in those suffering from anorexia nervosa and that metoclopramide can relieve this. Seven patients were treated with metoclopramide 10 mg four times daily for one month and gained between 1.8 and 8.1 kg in weight. In addition there was a noticeable overall improvement in symptoms such as intolerance of meals, epigastric pain after eating, excessive belching, vomiting, anorexia, and early satiety. No side-effects were noted, but it did not relieve anxiety as some patients were frightened by their weight gain and stopped treatment. Bethanicol and domperidone have also been shown to accelerate gastric emptying in anorexia nervosa, but their value in treating this disorder has yet to be established (Dubois, Gross and Ebert, 1980; Russell *et al.*, 1983).

Opiate antagonists

Having failed to achieve any success with drugs which blocked neurotransmission such as noradrenaline, acetylcholine, dopamine or serotonin, Mills investigated the effect of naloxone (Moore, Mills and Forster, 1981). A recent report concerns 10 patients who received between 1.6 and 6.4 mg daily for a period ranging from 19 to 61 days (Mills and Medlicott, 1984). They were also given amitriptyline and anticonvulsants and were encouraged to take a 3000 kcal diet. Marked increases in weight occurred and eight patients were reported as being in excellent health when reviewed 6 months later. This effect was attributed both to naloxone's antilipolytic actions and its blocking of opiate-determined compulsive behaviour. Unfortunately, this treatment is very expensive and has to be given by continuous intravenous infusion.

Zinc

Thomsen (1978) was probably the first to suggest that zinc deficiency may play a part in the pathogenesis of anorexia nervosa. He proposed that an inadequate intake of zinc could result in nausea and so worsen the aversion for food, thereby setting up a vicious circle. Bakan (1979) and Horrobin and Cunnane (1980) supported this view and drew attention to the similarities between anorexia nervosa and the zinc-deficiency syndrome, Bakan emphasizing that adolescent girls who diet are especially likely to become lacking in zinc. Safai-Kutti and Kutti (1984) and Bryce-Smith and Simpson (1984a) then reported single cases of anorexia nervosa in whom oral zinc sulphate resulted in a marked increase in appetite and weight. Bryce-Smith and Simpson (1984b) advocated giving zinc to those anorectics who are unable to taste a 1.0% solution of zinc sulphate. There have been reports of a few similar patients, but as yet there has been no double-blind trial (Bryce-Smith, 1986; Safai-Kutti and Kutti, 1986). Three of our patients with low serum zinc levels received oral zinc sulphate in addition to neuroleptics and insulin. Two discharged themselves before their response could be evaluated, and the third fared no better than on the occasions she was treated without zinc supplements.

Summary

Many medical measures have been used in the management of this disorder but none has proved universally effective. When they have produced weight gain it is not always clear why, and their apparent success has not always stood up to further scrutiny. Our preference is for the use of a combination of moderate doses of neuroleptics and insulin, and this is described in the next chapter.

References

ALTSHULER, K. Z. and WEINER, M. F. (1985) Anorexia nervosa and depression: a dissenting view. *Am. J. Psychiatry*, **142**, 328–332

References

ANDERSEN, M. S. (1928) Insulin som understotteles-middel ved fedekure. *Ugeskr. Laeger*, **90**, 1013–1017

BAKAN, R. (1979) The role of zinc in anorexia nervosa: etiology and treatment. *Med. Hypotheses*, **5**, 731–736

BARCAI, A. (1977) Lithium in adult anorexia nervosa: a pilot report on two patients. *Acta Psychiatr. Scand.*, **55**, 97–101

BARRY, V. C. and KLAWANS, H. L. (1976) On the role of dopamine in the pathophysiology of anorexia nervosa. *J. Neural Transm.*, **38**, 107–122

BEMIS, K. M. (1978) Current approaches to the etiology and treatment of anorexia nervosa. *Psychol. Bull.*, **85**, 593–617

BENADY, D. R. (1970) Cyproheptadine hydrochloride (Periactin) and anorexia nervosa: a case report. *Br. J. Psychiatry*, **117**, 681–682

BHANJI, S. (1979) Anorexia nervosa: physicians' and psychiatrists' opinions and practice. *J. Psychosom. Res.*, **23**, 7–11

BIEDERMAN, J., HERZOG, D. B., RIVINUS, T. M., HARPER, G. P., FERBER, R. A., ROSENBAUM, J. F. *et al.* (1985) Amitriptyline in the treatment of anorexia nervosa: a double-blind placebo-controlled study. *J. Clin. Psychopharmacol.*, **5**, 10–16

BOND, D. D. (1949) Anorexia nervosa. *Rocky Mountain Med. J.*, **46**, 1012–1019

BRYCE-SMITH, D. (1986) Environmental chemical influences on behaviour and mentation. *Chem. Soc. Rev.*, **15**, 99–123

BRYCE-SMITH, D. and SIMPSON, R. I. D. (1984a) Case of anorexia nervosa responding to zinc sulphate. *Lancet*, ii, 350

BRYCE-SMITH, D. and SIMPSON, R. I. D. (1984b) Anorexia, depression, and zinc deficiency. *Lancet*, ii, 1162

CLOW, F. E. (1932) Anorexia nervosa. *New Engl. J. Med.*, **207**, 613–617

CRISP, A. H. (1965) Clinical and therapeutic aspects of anorexia nervosa—a study of 30 cases. *J. Psychosom. Res.*, **9**, 67–77

CRISP, A. H. (1984) Treatment of anorexia nervosa: what can be the role of psychopharmacological agents? In *The Psychobiology of Anorexia Nervosa*, edited by K. M. Pirke and D. Ploog, pp. 148–160. Berlin: Springer-Verlag

DALLY, P. (1981) Treatment of anorexia nervosa. *Br. J. Hosp. Med.*, **25**, 434–440

DALLY, P. J., OPPENHEIM, G. B. and SARGANT, W. (1958) Anorexia nervosa. *Br. Med. J.*, ii, 633–634

DOLECEK, R. and JANSTOVA, V. (1985) Long-term effect of pizotifen treatment on growth hormone levels of underweight children, including those with anorexia nervosa. *Pharmatherapeutica*, **4**, 81–87

DUBOIS, A., GROSS, H. A. and EBERT, W. H. (1980) Bethanechol stimulated gastric emptying and acid output in anorexia nervosa patients. *Dig. Dis. Sci.*, **25**, 716

FINKELSTEIN, B. A. (1972) Parenteral hyperalimentation in anorexia nervosa. *J. Am. Med. Assoc.*, **219**, 217

GOLDBERG, S. C., HALMI, K. A., ECKERT, E. D., CASPER, R. C. and DAVIS, J. M. (1979) Cyproheptadine in anorexia nervosa. *Br. J. Psychiatry*, **134**, 67–70

GREEN, R. S. and RAU, J. H. (1977) The use of diphenylhydantoin in compulsive eating disorders: further studies. In: *Anorexia Nervosa*, edited by R. A. Vigorsky, pp. 377–382. New York: Raven Press

GROSS, H., EBERT, M. H., FADEN, V. B., GOLDBERG, S. C., KAYE, W. H., CAINE, E. D. *et al.* (1983) A double-blind trial of delta-9-tetrahydrocannabinol in primary anorexia nervosa. *J. Clin. Psychopharmacol.*, **3**, 165–171

GROSS, H. A., EBERT, M. H., FADEN, V. B., GOLDBERG, S. C., NEE, L. E. and KAYE, W. H. (1981) A double-blind controlled trial of lithium carbonate in primary anorexia nervosa. *J. Clin. Psychopharmacol.*, **1**, 376–381

HALMI, K. A., ECKERT, E., LODU, T. J. and COHEN, J. (1986) Anorexia nervosa: treatment efficacy of cyproheptadine and amitriptyline. *Arch. Gen. Psychiatry*, **43**, 177–181

HARRIS, B., YOUNG, J. and HUGHES, B. (1986) Comparative effects of seven antidepressant regimes on appetite, weight and carbohydrate preference. *Br. J. Psychiatry*, **148**, 590–592

HARROWER, A. D. B., YAP, P. L., NAIRN, I. M., WALTON, H. J., STRONG, J. A. and CRAIG, A. (1977) Growth hormone, insulin, and prolactin secretion in anorexia nervosa and obesity during bromocriptine treatment. *Br. Med. J.*, ii, 156–159

HIRSCHMAN, G. H., RAO, D. D. and CHAN, J. C. M. (1977) Anorexia nervosa with acute tubular necrosis treated with parenteral nutrition. *Nutr. Metab.*, **21**, 341–348

HORROBIN, D. F. and CUNNANE, S. C. (1980) Interactions between zinc, essential fatty acids and prostaglandins: relevance to acrodermatitis enteropathica, total parenteral nutrition, the glucagonoma syndrome, diabetes, anorexia nervosa and sickle cell anaemia. *Med. Hypotheses*, **6**, 277–296

HUDSON, J. I., POPE, H. G., JONAS, J. M. and YURGELUN-TODD, D. (1985) Treatment of anorexia with antidepressants. *J. Clin. Psychopharmacol.*, **5**, 17–23

JOHANSON, A. J. and KNORR, N. J. (1977) L-dopa as treatment for anorexia nervosa. In *Anorexia Nervosa*, edited by R. Vigorsky, pp. 363–372. New York: Raven Press

JOHNSON, C., STUCKEY, M. and MITCHELL, J. (1983) Psychopharmacological treatment of anorexia nervosa and bulimia. *J. Nerv. Ment. Dis.*, **171**, 524–534

KENNEDY, S. H., PIRAN, N. and GARFINKEL, P. E. (1985) Monoamine oxidase inhibitor therapy for anorexia nervosa and bulimia: a preliminary trial of isocarboxazid. *J. Clin. Psychopharmacol.*, **5**, 279–285

KERRY, R. J., LIEBLING, L. I. and OWEN, G. (1970) Weight changes in lithium responders. *Acta Psychiatr. Scand.*, **46**, 238–243

LACEY, J. H. and CRISP, A. H. (1980) Hunger, food intake and weight: the impact of clomipramine on a refeeding anorexia nervosa population. *Postgrad. Med. J.*, **56**, 79–85

MCCULLAGH, E. P. and TUPPER, W. R. (1940) Anorexia nervosa. *Ann. Int. Med.*, **14**, 817–838

MALONEY, M. J. and FARRELL, M. K. (1980) Treatment of severe weight loss in anorexia nervosa with hyperalimentation and psychotherapy. *Am. J. Psychiatry*, **137**, 310–314

MAWSON, A. R. (1974) Anorexia nervosa and the regulation of intake: a review. *Psychol. Med.*, **4**, 289–308

MILLS, I. H. and MEDLICOTT, L. (1984) The basis of naloxone treatment in anorexia nervosa and the metabolic responses to it. In *The Psychobiology of Anorexia Nervosa*, edited by K. M. Pirke and D. Ploog, pp. 161–171. Berlin: Springer-Verlag

MOORE, R., MILLS, I. H. and FORSTER, A. (1981) Naloxone in the treatment of anorexia nervosa: effect on weight gain and lipolysis. *J. R. Soc. Med.*, **74**, 129–131

PAYKEL, E. S., MUELLER, P. S. and DE LA VERGNE, P. M. (1973) Amitriptyline, weight gain and carbohydrate craving: a side effect. *Br. J. Psychiatry*, **123**, 501–507

PERTSCHUK, M. J., FORSTER, J., BUZBY, G. and MULLEN, J. L. (1981) The treatment of anorexia nervosa with total parenteral nutrition. *Biol. Psychiatry*, **16**, 539–550

PLANTEY, F. (1977) Pimozide in treatment of anorexia nervosa. *Lancet*, i, 1105

RAU, J. H., STRUVE, F. A. and GREEN, R. S. (1979) Electroencephalographic correlates of compulsive eating. *Clin. Electroencephalogr.*, **10**, 180–188

REDMOND, D. E., SWANN, A. and HENINGER, G. R. (1976) Phenoxybenzamine in anorexia nervosa. *Lancet*, ii, 307

RUSSELL, D. MCR., FREEDMAN, M. L., FEIGHLIN, D. H. I., JEEJEEBOY, K. N., SWINSON, R. P. and GARFINKEL, P. E. (1983) Delayed gastric emptying and improvement with domperidone in a patient with anorexia nervosa. *Am. J. Psychiatry*, **140**, 1235–1236

RUSSELL, G. F. M. (1985) Do drugs have a place in the management of anorexia nervosa and bulimia nervosa. In *Psychopharmacology and Food*, edited by M. Sandler and T. Silverstone, pp. 146–161. Oxford: Oxford University Press

RYLE, J. A. (1936) Anorexia nervosa. *Lancet*, ii, 893–899

SAFAI-KUTTI, S. and KUTTI, J. (1984) Zinc and anorexia nervosa. *Ann. Int. Med.*, **100**, 317–318

SAFAI-KUTTI, S. and KUTTI, J. (1986) Zinc supplementation in anorexia nervosa. *Am. J. Clin. Nutr.*, **44**, 581–582

SALEH, J. W. and LEBWOHL, P. (1980) Metoclopramide-induced gastric emptying in patients with anorexia nervosa. *Am. J. Gastroenterol.*, **74**, 127–132

THOMSEN, K. (1978) Zinc, liver cirrhosis and anorexia nervosa. *Acta Derm. Venereol.*, **58**, 283

VANDEREYCKEN, W. (1984) Neuroleptics in the short-term treatment of anorexia nervosa: a double-blind placebo-controlled study with sulpiride. *Br. J. Psychiatry*, **144**, 288–292

VANDEREYCKEN, W. and PIERLOOT, R. (1982) Pimozide combined with behavior therapy in the short-term treatment of anorexia nervosa. *Acta Psychiatr. Scand.*, **66**, 445–450

VIGERSKY, R. A. and LORIAUX, D. L. (1977) The effect of cyproheptadine in anorexia nervosa: a double-blind trial. In *Anorexia Nervosa*, edited by R. A. Vigersky, pp. 349–356. New York: Raven Press

WERMUTH, B. M., DAVIS, K. L., HOLLISTER, L. E. and STUNKARD, A. J. (1977) Phenytoin treatment of the binge-eating syndrome. *Am. J. Psychiatry*, **134**, 1249–1253

WILLIAMS, E. (1958) Anorexia nervosa: a somatic disorder. *Br. Med. J.*, ii, 190–195

YOUNG, J. K. (1975) A possible neuroendocrine basis of two clinical syndromes: anorexia nervosa and the Kleine-Levin syndrome. *Physiol. Psychol.*, **3**, 322–330

Chapter 16

The authors' management regimen

The various forms of medical and psychiatric management have been discussed in the previous chapters. This chapter concentrates on treatment with neuroleptics and insulin, and presents the authors' regimen.

Sargant and his colleagues at St Thomas's Hospital, London, were the first to describe a treatment for anorexia nervosa which involved the use of insulin and chlorpromazine, in addition to admission to hospital for bed rest and supervised meals (Dally, Oppenheim and Sargant, 1958). Their starting dose of insulin was 5–10 units and the maximum daily dosage up to 80 units. Chlorpromazine was started at the same time as the insulin, the initial dose ranging from 150–300 mg/day. The average duration of treatment was 36 days and the mean weight gain was 10.4 kg at a mean rate of 0.3 kg each day. The amount and rate of weight gain were greater than in patients treated with insulin alone or just by bed rest (Dally and Sargant, 1960, 1966). Severe side-effects were not uncommon and some 15% of their patients had convulsions due either to hypoglycaemia or the toxic effects of the chlorpromazine. The use of neuroleptics and insulin in the treatment of anorexia nervosa has therefore fallen out of favour. Nevertheless, we believe that both can play a valuable role, providing that only modest doses are used and that stringent steps are taken to avoid side-effects. We also believe that the anorectic can be treated successfully on a general medical ward without recourse to traditional means such as insistence on bed rest and supervised high calorie meals, and formal psychiatric treatment. We do not claim to cure the illness, but to induce a fairly rapid remission. In many of our patients this has so far proved lasting, and in others it has enabled psychotherapy to be started or resumed with success.

Patients

From February 1975 to April 1986, 87 patients suffering from anorexia nervosa were admitted for treatment to an acute medical ward of a district general hospital.

In keeping with the sex distribution of the illness, all but two cases were female. Their ages on admission ranged from 13 to 67 years (mean 21.4 years). The time since commencement of weight loss varied from 3 months to 20 years (mean 32.8 months). Thirty-three patients had been ill for at least 2 years, and 29 had habitually abused laxatives or made themselves vomit. The weight on admission lay between 26.6 and 59.5 kg (mean 39.1 kg). This represented from 46 to 90% (mean 70%) of the optimum for the sex, age and height of the patient.

Management

Most of the patients were nursed in six-bedded bays, a few in cubicles. As previous experience had taught that a too coercive or restrictive approach is likely to provoke early self-discharge, the intention from the outset was that the anorectics should be treated as any other patient admitted to the ward. Hence bed rest was not insisted upon unless medically necessary. The anorectics were allowed a free choice from the ward menu, and meals were not supervised. The nurses, however, would report if food had been returned. Similarly, although no steps were taken to prevent or penalize deliberate postprandial vomiting, its occurrence was noted. There were no restrictions on visiting, correspondence or gifts, and brief outings were encouraged during the latter part of the patients' stay in hospital.

A target weight for discharge was decided on admission. The patients were expected to reach 90% of their calculated optimum weight. The target was not usually disclosed immediately to those who were grossly underweight or apprehensive about staying in hospital. The patients were weighed daily after breakfast, and a graphical record kept. This was used to illustrate progress to the patient and relatives, and provided an invaluable guide as to the effectiveness of treatment. Because of the difficulties and disadvantages of keeping young, active people in hospital and the demand for acute medical beds, some patients were discharged before reaching their target. This occurred only where weight was being regained at a steady rate and the patient's attitude and behaviour gave grounds for optimism.

Most cases were seen by a psychiatrist to exclude those mental illnesses such as depression, schizophrenia and obsessional neurosis which may be associated with poor appetite or perverse eating habits. Advice was given as to the risk of suicide in those who felt depressed, and counselling was available to those who wished to discuss emotional or social problems.

Chlorpromazine was the most commonly used neuroleptic and was given as an elixir in order to minimize surreptitious disposal and to permit easy dose increments. The dosage was increased in stepwise fashion, often from as little as 10 mg three times daily, to a maximum which ranged from 60 to 1000 mg/day (mean 283 mg). This was determined largely by the tolerance of the patient, the commonest side-effects being drowsiness and mild extrapyramidal symptoms. A number of patients received another neuroleptic, pimozide, as crushed tablets. At first pimozide was prescribed only to those unable to tolerate chlorpromazine. Later both drugs were given together as it was found that a combination of low dosages of each was equally effective and produced less drowsiness. The maximum daily dose of pimozide ranged from 1 to 16 mg (mean 5.5 mg). Two girls who developed a fall in the white cell count while on chlorpromazine were given haloperidol instead.

Insulin was usually started 2 or 3 days after the neuroleptic. The initial dose consisted of only two units of purified porcine or synthetic human insulin given subcutaneously after breakfast. Thereafter it was given before lunch and supper as well, the total daily dose being slowly increased by two units a day until a steady weight gain was observed. The maximum daily dose rarely exceeded 30 units. Special care was taken to avoid hypoglycaemia in the early stages of treatment for it was found that as little as two units of insulin could produce it in some of the emaciated patients. Blood glucose levels were monitored by the nursing staff, using BM glycaemic sticks, and the next injection of insulin was omitted if the level was below 4 mmol/l. Once the patients began to put on weight this precaution was no longer necessary.

As regards other medication, three depressed patients were prescribed antidepressants, and three epileptics continued to receive their anticonvulsants. Antibiotics were required by five patients who developed chest infections. Metoclopramide was given to five patients who complained of marked nausea but we did not find it effective, and one girl who was also taking chlorpromazine developed marked orofacial dystonia after a single dose of 10 mg. Four patients developed ankle oedema during a period of rapid weight gain and were given a short course of frusemide. Finally, nine were prescribed orphenadrine or procyclidine for extrapyramidal side-effects.

Results

Of the 87 patients admitted for treatment 10 discharged themselves prematurely against advice, one left hospital after only 10 days of treatment in order to be with her family over Christmas and refused readmission, and one had to be transferred to a

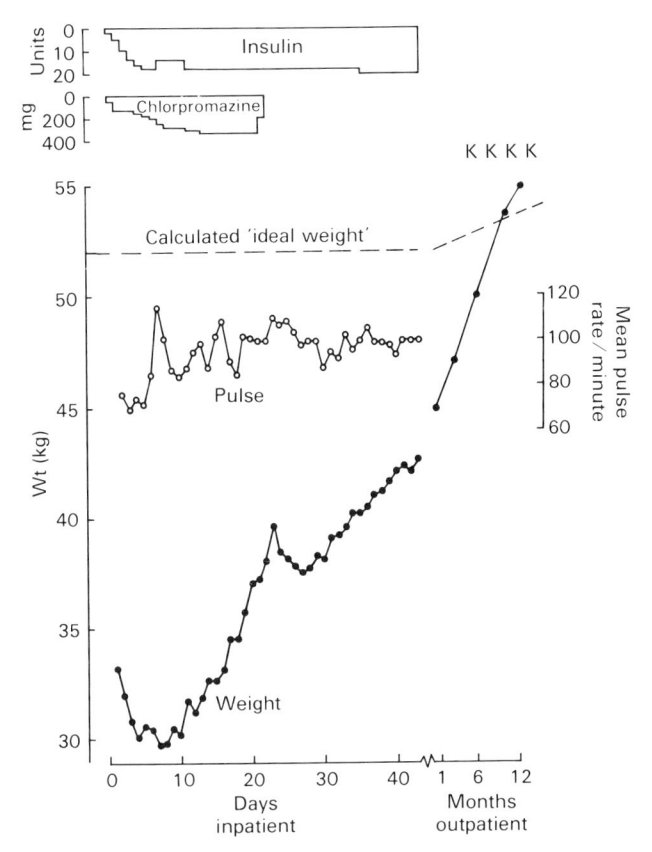

Figure 16.1 Response to treatment in a 15-year-old girl with primary amenorrhoea whose weight had fallen to 63% of her premorbid weight over the previous year. After a latent period of about 10 days she put on weight rapidly until the chlorpromazine was stopped when she developed a photosensitivity rash. After 3 days she began to put on weight again on insulin alone, though at a slower rate than on the combined treatment. She was discharged from hospital when her weight was 82% of her calculated optimum. Ten months later this had risen to 99% and she had started to menstruate regularly

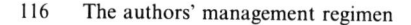

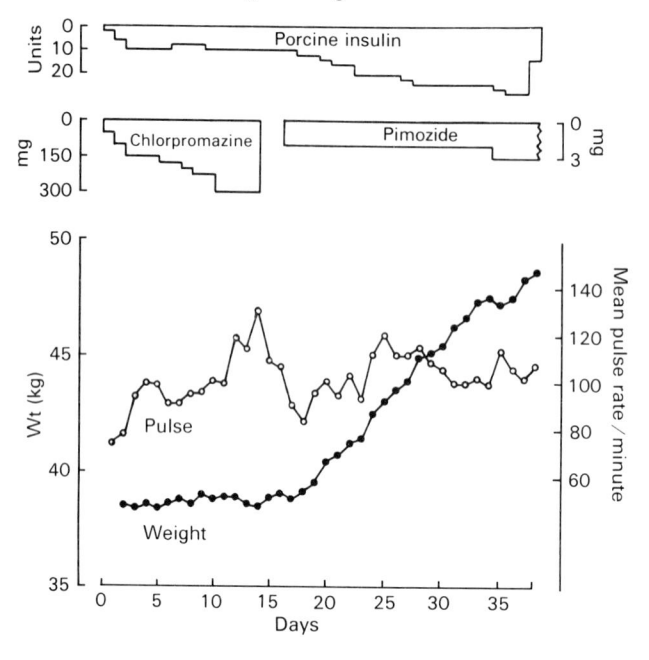

Figure 16.2 Response to treatment in a 14-year-old girl with secondary amenorrhoea whose weight had fallen to about 60% of the calculated optimum in 5 months. After 2 weeks she developed a fever, tachycardia and disturbed liver function tests which were thought to be due to chlorpromazine hypersensitivity. These abnormalities disappeared when this drug was stopped and replaced by pimozide. Shortly afterwards she began to gain weight rapidly and left hospital at 81% of her calculated optimum weight. She later relapsed and was admitted for a further course of treatment

psychiatric hospital following a carefully planned attempt at suicide. These 12 patients, all but three of whom had been ill for at least 5 years, will not be considered further.

The 75 patients who stayed in hospital received treatment over a period ranging from 12 to 118 days (mean 41 days). When discharged all except four had shown satisfactory weight gains. These four patients consisted of three chronic anorectics and a younger patient with considerable family problems.

The progress of the 71 patients whom we regard as having responded to treatment is now discussed. Although 11 patients began to regain weight as soon as treatment was started, this was unusual. In the majority there was a latent period of 2–50 days (mean 13 days), during which a weight loss of 1–2 kg was not uncommon. The mean latent period was shorter in the vomiters and purgers (8.7 days) than in the dieters (15.3 days), this difference being statistically significant ($P<0.05$). There was no correlation, however, between the length of the latent period and the chronicity of the illness.

The growth period, during which weight was regained, lasted from 7 to 65 days (mean 28.8 days) and was often preceded by an abrupt rise in the resting pulse rate (*Figures 16.1–16.3*). The mean weight gain during this growth period was 9.8 kg and ranged from 4.2 to 20.8 kg, at an average rate of between 0.12 and 0.91 kg/day (mean 0.38 kg/day). The rate at which the weight increased tended to be higher in those who had been ill for less than 2 years and also in those who induced vomiting or took large

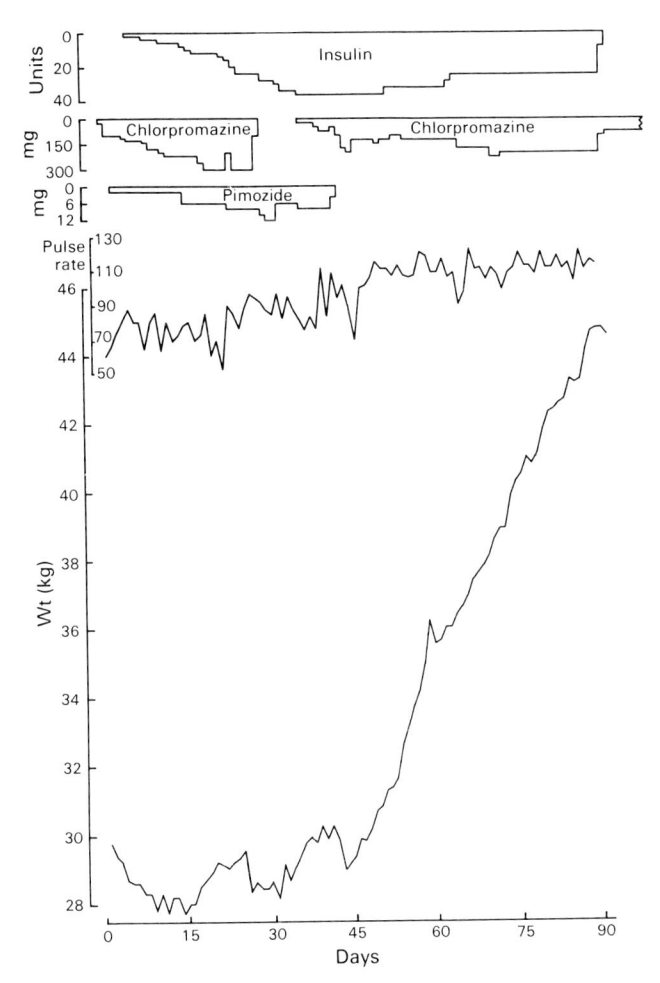

Figure 16.3 Response to treatment in a tall 14-year-old girl with secondary amenorrhoea whose weight had fallen to 50% of her calculated optimum in less than 6 months. There was an exceptionally long latent period during which she had several hypoglycaemic reactions and developed micrographia and extrapyramidal signs necessitating a reduction in dosage. The period of rapid weight gain was heralded by a sustained rise in her pulse rate and she left hospital at 78% of her calculated optimum weight. Ten months later this had risen to 97% and she was menstruating regularly. She was still in remission 5 years later

amounts of laxatives. These differences were not statistically significant. The mean discharge weight was 87% of the optimum.

As well as the obvious improvement in the patients' physical state, there were noticeable psychological changes. Many patients lost their fear of becoming obese, once it was explained that this had rarely happened to our other cases and that their target weight was by no means excessive. In most of those who complained of depression when admitted there was an apparently spontaneous improvement in mood and morale once weight gain was well under way. Furthermore, the morose and withdrawn would often become charming and self-assured, and the sullenly reticent

Table 16.1 Side-effects of treatment in 54 patients

Side-effects	%
Drowsiness	48
Extrapyramidal symptoms	39
Mild hypoglycaemic symptoms	24
Ankle oedema	11
Skin rash	11
Giddiness	9
Blurring of vision	4
Convulsions	4
Fall in blood white cell count	4
Headache	2
Pyrexia	2
Sore mouth	2

more willing to discuss their problems. All this happened without any specific psychiatric measures.

Side-effects of treatment were seen in 54 patients (*Table 16.1*). The commonest were drowsiness, extrapyramidal symptoms and mild hypoglycaemia. Most of the side-effects attributable to the neuroleptics could be dealt with by reduction of the dosage or, in nine cases by an antiparkinsonian drug. The most frequent extrapyramidal side-effect was mild rigidity which was usually noticed early by the nursing staff. An interesting finding was the development of micrographia in two cases. All patients on chlorpromazine were warned to avoid direct sunlight because of the risk of photosensitivity dermatitis, and the use of a barrier cream appeared to minimize this potential complication. In the six cases who developed a rash the drug was stopped. The other indication for stopping or changing neuroleptic therapy was a fall in the white cell count.

Follow-up

Thirty-nine (55%) of the 71 patients described above were followed-up by one or both of us for at least 12 months, the longest period being 6 years. At the end of this time only four patients were still receiving medication. Three were on small doses of a neuroleptic and one was taking an antidepressant. During the follow-up period 19 patients relapsed, and 17 agreed to come back into hospital for a further course of treatment. One young woman, a vomiter and purger, who had been anorectic for 5 years required five admissions before she went into a remission which so far has lasted well over 4 years. No significant difference between the relapsers and the rest could be shown with respect to the severity or duration of the illness on first presentation, the dosage of drugs required or the initial response to treatment, nor did the relapsers contain a significantly higher proportion of vomiters or purgers.

When last seen the mean weight of all 39 patients was 91% of the optimum, readjusted where necessary to allow for increased age and height. Twenty-five patients (66%) were eating normally, without obvious or expressed anxiety. Their weights ranged from 74 to 115% of the optimum, being above 90% in 15. Fourteen had resumed menstruation spontaneously. Twelve remained preoccupied with their diet and seven of these patients were still more than 10% underweight. Two of these were binging and then inducing vomiting, and only two were menstruating. Finally, two patients were clearly obese, but only one was having periods. In keeping with the findings of others, those with the shorter histories before being treated fared better than those who had been ill for more than 2 years.

Discussion

Although we agree with the longheld view that admission to hospital is often necessary, our experience suggests that insistence on strict bed rest, supervised high calorie meals, punishments and rewards, and the early setting of an inflexible target weight are not essential prerequisites for a successful outcome.

The beneficial results of our treatment are comparable to those of Dally and Sargant (1966) who were the first to advocate the combination of chlorpromazine and insulin in the treatment of anorexia nervosa. However, the regimen we describe differs from theirs in many respects, particularly with regard to dosage. Our results suggest that in many cases relatively low doses of neuroleptics will suffice, with a consequent reduction in serious side-effects. Like Dally and Sargant we had previously found that patients treated with neuroleptics and insulin together gained weight faster than when on either alone. We employed smaller amounts of insulin as the intention was not to produce hypoglycaemia, and hence hunger, but to encourage the rapid replacement of fat in the depleted adipose tissues. Anorectic patients are very vulnerable to small doses of insulin, as little as two units producing hypoglycaemia in some of our cases. Hence the advantage of treating these patients on a general medical ward where the medical and nursing staff are familiar with the observation and management of the young insulin-dependent diabetic.

Both staff and patients need to be aware of the latent period and should not be disheartened if weight gain does not occur within the first week or two. This delay is in keeping with that seen when the neuroleptics are used to treat psychoses, but the mode of action of these drugs in anorexia nervosa has yet to be established. However, it may be relevant that they are dopamine antagonists.

A major fear of the patient being treated for anorexia nervosa is that the outcome will be loss of control over the appetite. When last seen only two of our cases were binging and only two were more than 15% above their calculated optimum weight. It is also commonly noted that the successful resolution of anorexia nervosa may be followed by depression. Only five patients required antidepressant medication after leaving hospital and all had been depressed before their admission. Only one was still taking an antidepressant when last seen. Over half the patients we were able to follow-up appear to have gone into remission after one course of treatment, and many of those who relapsed eventually responded. Although the relapse rate was disappointing it was not entirely unexpected, for similar results have been reported following other forms of treatment.

Summary

Treatment with small doses of neuroleptics and insulin in an acute medical ward seems to be as successful as many other methods that have been described. It has the advantages of being relatively brief, non-coercive, and without the regrettable stigmata attached to admission to a mental hospital. We publish our experience in treating this disorder in the hope that it will encourage more physicians to take an active interest in these unfortunate girls. We believe that in many cases their efforts will be well rewarded.

References

DALLY, P. and SARGANT, W. (1966) Treatment and outcome of anorexia nervosa. *Br. Med. J.*, ii, 793–795
DALLY, P. J., OPPENHEIM, G. B. and SARGANT, W. (1958) Anorexia nervosa. *Br. Med. J.*, ii, 633–634
DALLY, P. J. and SARGANT, W. (1960) A new treatment for anorexia nervosa. *Br. Med. J.*, i, 1770–1772.

Chapter 17

Prognosis

Opinions on the long-term outcome of anorexia nervosa have varied widely ever since the earliest descriptions. The first of Morton's cases, Miss Duke, died after being ill for some time (Morton, 1689). In contrast Gull (1874) regarded the outlook as good, although he did mention one fatal case, and Lasegue (1873) described the prognosis as always favourable. More recent reports suggested that anorexia nervosa is a serious illness with significant chronic morbidity and mortality (Kay and Leigh, 1954; Williams, 1958). Other writers have emphasized the marked variability in outcome (Crisp, 1965; Morgan and Russell, 1975; Garfinkel, Moldofsky and Garner, 1977; Hsu, Crisp and Harding, 1979).

The immediate response to treatment is usually good, especially where weight correction is the major criterion. The rate at which this is achieved tends to be slow in methods relying heavily on individual psychotherapy, but noticeably faster with medical or behavioural approaches (Blinder, Freeman and Stunkard, 1970). The type of treatment given, however, appears to have little bearing in the long-term (Morgan and Russell, 1975; Crisp et al., 1977; Russell, 1977).

Methodology

The assessment of the long-term results of treatment are bedevilled by methodological problems. These have been reviewed recently by Hsu (1980), Schwartz and Thompson (1981), and Steinhausen and Glanville (1983). Major difficulties in the interpretation of studies of outcome arise out of the inconstant ways in which anorexia nervosa has been defined, and the measures of successful treatment chosen and recorded. Even such an objective sign of progress as weight is often expressed loosely as 'low', 'normal' or 'overweight'. Similarly, if menstrual status is reported there is seldom any reference to the frequency, regularity or amount of bleeding. Emotive topics such as eating habits and psychological adjustment may be deliberately misreported by the informant, although matters such as occupational and marital status can be more reliably assessed. Many studies have been based on case records, which may be inaccurate or incomplete, or on postal or telephone enquiries to the family doctor or another hospital. Very few follow-up surveys have involved a standardized, independent and personal reassessment of the patient herself.

The duration of follow-up is also important; a short period of observation has the advantage that cases may be easier to trace, but is more likely to include patients who have yet to relapse. A prolonged follow-up may include cases who have received other treatment elsewhere. A final problem is one of selection bias. Most of the larger-scale studies have been conducted from centres with a known special interest in anorexia nervosa. Hence, it could be argued that they tend to see particularly difficult patients who are therefore less likely to do well (Morgan, Purgold and Wellbourne, 1983).

Morgan and Russell (1975) laid down the conditions they believed necessary for an adequate follow-up study. First, the patients should be consecutive cases treated in the same manner by the same consultant. Standardized criteria should be adopted so far as diagnosis, the features under investigation, and the outcome measures are concerned. Whenever possible the patients should be assessed personally by the same person, and the information corroborated independently. The minimum follow-up period should be 4 years. Finally, no case should be left unaccounted for.

These conditions are extremely difficult to achieve in clinical practice and have seldom been met. Nevertheless, those studies with lengthy follow-up periods have tended to produce similar findings in spite of considerable differences in methodology. About 40% of anorectics are totally recovered, 30% will have improved, and 30% have either died or remained chronically ill. So far as specific features of the illness are concerned, the outcome in terms of body weight is better than that regarding menstruation; this in turn is more satisfactory than psychological adjustment (Hsu, 1980).

Age of onset

It is widely believed that the younger the patient is when she develops the illness the better is the prognosis. The favourable effect of an early age of onset has been demonstrated in a number of studies. Some, by contrast, have found that this bears no relationship to the long-term outlook, and Swift (1982) and Hawley (1985) have criticized the evidence linking an early onset with a good prognosis. Furthermore, Dally (1969) expected the outcome to be poor if the illness developed before the age of 14 years. Morgan and Russell (1975) found that the age at which weight loss began did not correlate with either a good or a poor eventual outcome, but if the illness was dated from the onset of amenorrhoea a later onset was followed by a worse prognosis. Whether or not the amenorrhoea antedated the fall in weight had no influence. Halmi et al. (1979) reported that the age at which their patients became ill was bimodally distributed, with peaks at 14.5 and 18 years. The possibility that age alone may not be an important prognostic indicator was raised by the finding that the older group had a number of other features thought to indicate a poor prognosis.

Weight loss

Ever since Morton (1689) suggested that the sooner the doctor be called in the better, there has been almost unanimous support for the view that a short duration of weight loss augurs well for the future. However, Browning and Miller (1968) and Nussbaum et al. (1985) failed to demonstrate any correlation between this and the ultimate prognosis. There is also disagreement over the significance of the extent of weight loss. Some have shown that the prognosis is poorer in those who have lost more weight, but others report that this is not so and this has been our experience. There is a consensus that binging, self-induced vomiting and the abuse of purgatives or diuretics carry a worse prognosis. Our patients who lost weight mainly because of vomiting or purging were more likely to refuse treatment, but those who accepted did just as well as our dieters.

Demographic factors

As male cases of primary anorexia are probably even rarer than is usually stated (Beumont, Beardwood and Russell, 1972) it is difficult to draw any firm conclusions regarding the effect of sex on prognosis. Crisp et al. (1977) and Dally (1969) regarded the prognosis as being poorer in males, but the three males followed up by Morgan and Russell (1975) had all done well. Tolstrup et al. (1985) found no difference in outcome between the two sexes, but the males were significantly younger.

Being married would appear to carry a poor prognosis (Seidensticker and Tzagournis, 1968; Crisp et al., 1977; Hsu, Crisp and Harding, 1979; Hall et al., 1984), although Halmi, Brodland and Loney (1973) found that their single and married subjects fared equally well. Social class and occupational attainment probably have little, if any, effect on prognosis (Seidensticker and Tzagournis, 1968; Theander, 1970; Morgan and Russell, 1975; Pierloot, Wellens and Houben, 1975; Morgan, Purgold and Wellbourne, 1983). There are some studies, nevertheless, which present the contrary view and suggest that patients from the lower classes do less well (Halmi, Brodland and Loney, 1973; Crisp et al., 1977; Hsu, Crisp and Harding, 1979), perhaps because they and their families are less willing or able to cooperate with treatment (Kalucy, Crisp and Harding, 1977). Religious affiliation does not appear to influence long-term progress (Seidensticker and Tzagournis, 1968).

Birth complications

Morgan and Russell (1975) reported that there was no apparent connection between birth complications and either a good or a bad prognosis. This is in contrast to the finding of Halmi et al. (1979) that problematical deliveries were associated with a history of a poor response to previous hospital treatment, and the view that there is a subgroup of anorectics with minimal neurological deficits who respond less well to treatment (Hamsher, Halmi and Benton, 1981). Theander (1970) found that patients born to older mothers fared less well, but this was not confirmed (Halmi, Brodland and Loney, 1973). Neither birth order (Seidensticker and Tzagournis, 1968) nor early bereavement (Halmi, Brodland and Loney, 1973) have been shown to affect prognosis.

Family background

An unusual family structure appears not to influence outcome (Morgan and Russell, 1975), but there is some doubt about the role of mental illness within the family. Morgan and Russell (1975) found this to be of little significance, but Crisp et al. (1977) and Kalucy, Crisp and Harding (1977) have between them described considerable family psychopathology which they claim is of prognostic as well as aetiological importance. A poor prognosis is associated with a high level of depression in the parents; in addition a high degree of obsessionality in the mother, a father who is preoccupied with somatic complaints, and a general over-concern about weight and body appearance are all said to bode ill.

A disturbed relationship between the anorectic and her parents may adversely affect progress after treatment (Morgan and Russell, 1975; Hsu, Crisp and Harding, 1979). Sibling rivalry probably has no influence on the prognosis. Theander (1970) and Pierloot, Wellens and Houben (1975), in contrast, did not find family relationships to have any prognostic value. As with most conditions with a psychological aspect, the premorbid personality plays a considerable part in determining the prognosis in anorexia nervosa. Those who do poorly have been described as either excessively conforming and compliant as children, or as being just the opposite (Morgan and Russell, 1975; Crisp et al., 1977; Hsu, Crisp and Harding, 1979; Morgan, Purgold and Wellbourne, 1983). Regarding later development, an inadequate or poorly adjusted personality is also likely to render the eventual outcome less than satisfactory (Ryle, 1939; Beck and Brochner-Mortensen, 1954; Morgan and Russell, 1975; Garfinkel, Moldofsky and Garner, 1977). However, Halmi, Brodland and Loney (1973) have not found this to be the case.

Precipitating factors

Although often of possible causal significance, an external precipitant appears not to have any influence on the prognosis (Theander, 1970; Halmi, Brodland and Loney, 1973; Morgan and Russell, 1975; Pierloot, Wellens and Houben, 1975). However, we find it difficult to believe that we are the only ones to observe that a relapse is more likely if the precipitant cannot be removed, alleviated, or come to terms with. Being teased about obesity is a common antecedent of anorexia nervosa, and Crisp et al. (1977) have noted premorbid obesity to be a sign of a poor prognosis. Morgan and Russell (1975) did not find this to be so, and Dally (1969) regarded mild obesity as a good sign.

Behavioural problems

Halmi, Brodland and Loney (1973) reported that the presence of depressive or obsessional behaviour indicates a poor prognosis, and Pierloot, Wellens and Houben (1975) made the same comment as regards stealing and self-mutilation. Garfinkel, Moldofsky and Garner (1977) found that overestimated body size usually indicated a poor long-term outlook. Anxiety when eating in front of others may be a further sign of a poor prognosis (Hsu, Crisp and Harding, 1979), and the persistence of morbid attitudes to eating may be associated with prolonged amenorrhoea, even if the weight is maintained at a reasonable level (Falk and Halmi, 1982).

Response to treatment

If a patient with anorexia nervosa has relapsed after previous treatment she is likely to do so again (Morgan and Russell, 1975; Hsu, Crisp and Harding, 1979; Morgan, Purgold and Wellbourne, 1983). Nevertheless, the immediate response to current therapy is thought to be of little prognostic significance. Browning and Miller (1968) found that the prognosis was not affected one way or the other by the amount of weight gained in hospital or the length of stay, and went so far as to question the need for admission as a matter of course.

Similarly Morgan and Russell (1975) and Pertschuk (1977) reported that the initial response to treatment did not serve to predict the later one. However, Beck and Brochner-Mortensen (1954) noted that a poor early response implied a poor outlook for the future, and Hsu, Crisp and Harding (1979) observed that a patient still doing well one year after discharge was more than likely to continue to do so.

Summary

This has been a chapter of at times confusing and contradictory guidance for the clinician. This is hardly surprising in view of the considerable methodological problems involved in the long-term study of a condition which is not only relatively rare among the general population, but is also poorly understood. In due course it may be demonstrated that physiological or biochemical factors provide a more reliable indicator of prognosis than clinical features and the personal background. In the meantime, the aphorism coined by our ward sister provides as good a guide as any: 'nice young girls from nice families do well'.

References

BECK, J. C. and BROCHNER-MORTENSEN, K. (1954) Observations on the prognosis of anorexia nervosa. *Acta Med. Scand.*, **149**, 409–430

BEUMONT, P. J. V., BEARDWOOD, C. J. and RUSSELL, G. F. M. (1972) The occurrence of the syndrome of anorexia nervosa on male subjects. *Psychol. Med.*, **2**, 216–231

BLINDER, B. J., FREEMAN, D. M. A. and STUNKARD, A. J. (1970) Behavior therapy of anorexia nervosa: effectiveness of activity as a reinforcer of weight gain. *Am J. Psychiatry*, **126**, 1093–1098

BROWNING, C. H. and MILLER, S. I. (1968) Anorexia nervosa: a study in prognosis and management. *Am. J. Psychiatry*, **124**, 1128–1132

CRISP, A. H. (1965) Some aspects of the evolution, presentation and follow-up of anorexia nervosa. *Proc. R. Soc. Med.*, **58**, 814–820

CRISP, A. H., KALUCY, R. S., LACEY, J. H. and HARDING, B. (1977) The long-term prognosis in anorexia nervosa: some factors predictive of outcome. In *Anorexia Nervosa*, edited by R. A. Vigersky, pp. 55–65. New York: Raven Press

DALLY, P. (1969) *Anorexia Nervosa*. London: William Heinemann Medical Books Ltd

FALK, J. R. and HALMI, K. A. (1882) Amenorrhea in anorexia nervosa: evaluation of the critical body weight hypothesis. *Biol. Psychiatry*, **17**, 799–806

GARFINKEL, P. E., MOLDOFSKY, H. and GARNER, D. M. (1977) Prognosis in anorexia nervosa as influenced by clinical features, treatment and self-perception. *Can. Med. Assoc. J.*, **117**, 1041–1045

GULL, W. W. (1874) Anorexia nervosa (apepsia hysterica, anorexia hysterica). *Trans. Clin. Soc. Lond.*, **7**, 22–28

HALL, A., SLIM, E., HAWKER, F. and SALMOND, C. (1984) Anorexia nervosa: long-term outcome in 50 female patients. *Br. J. Psychiatry*, **145**, 407–413

HALMI, K., BRODLAND, G. and LONEY, J. (1973) Prognosis in anorexia nervosa. *Ann. Intern. Med.*, **78**, 907–909

HALMI, K. A., CASPER, R. C., ECKERT, E. D., GOLDBERG, S. C. and DAVIS, J. M. (1979) Unique features associated with age of onset of anorexia nervosa. *Psychiatry Res.*, **1**, 209–215

HAMSHER, K. DE S., HALMI, K. A. and BENTON, A. L. (1981) Prediction in anorexia nervosa from neuropsychological status. *Psychiatry Res.*, **4**, 79–88

HAWLEY, R. M. (1985) The outcome of anorexia nervosa in younger subjects. *Br. J. Psychiatry*, **146**, 657–660

HSU, L. K. G. (1980) Outcome of anorexia nervosa: a review of the literature (1954 to 1978). *Arch. Gen. Psychiatry*, **37**, 1041–1046

HSU, L. K. G., CRISP, A. H. and HARDING, B. (1979) Outcome of anorexia nervosa. *Lancet*, i, 61–65

KALUCY, R. S., CRISP, A. H. and HARDING, B. (1977) A study of 56 families with anorexia nervosa. *Br. J. Med. Psychol.*, **50**, 381–395

KAY, D. W. K. and LEIGH, D. (1954) The natural history, treatment and prognosis of anorexia nervosa, based on a study of 38 patients. *J. Ment. Sci.*, **100**, 411–431

LASEGUE, C. (1873) De l'anorexie hysterique. *Arch. Gen. Med.*, **21**, 385–403

MORGAN, H. G., PURGOLD, J. and WELLBOURNE, J. (1983) Management and outcome in anorexia nervosa: a standardized prognostic study. *Br. J. Psychiatry*, **143**, 282–287

MORGAN, H. G. and RUSSELL, G. F. M. (1975) Value of family background and clinical features as predictors of long-term outcome in anorexia nervosa: four-year follow-up study of 41 patients. *Psychol. Med.*, **5**, 355–371

MORTON, R. (1689) *Phthisiologia: Sue exercitationes de phthisi*, pp. 4–11. London: S. Smith

NUSSBAUM, M., SHENKER, R., BAIRD, D. and SARAWAY, S. (1985) Follow-up investigation in patients with anorexia nervosa. *J. Pediatr.*, **106**, 835–840

PERTSCHUK, M. J. (1977) Behavior therapy: extended follow-up. In *Anorexia Nervosa*, edited by R. A. Vigersky, pp. 305–313. New York: Raven Press

PIERLOOT, R. A., WELLENS, W. and HOUBEN, M. E. (1975) Elements of resistance to a combined medical and psychotherapeutic program in anorexia nervosa. An overview. *Psychother. Psychosom.*, **26**, 101–117

RUSSELL, G. F. M. (1977) General management of anorexia nervosa and difficulties in assessing the efficacy of treatment. In *Anorexia Nervosa*, edited by R. A. Vigersky, pp. 277–290. New York: Raven Press

RYLE, J. A. (1939) Discussion on anorexia nervosa. *Proc. R. Soc. Med.*, **32**, 735–737

SCHWARTZ, D. M. and THOMPSON, M. G. (1981) Do anorexics get well? Current research and future needs. *Am. J. Psychiatry*, **138**, 319–323

SEIDENSTICKER, J. F. and TZAGOURNIS, M. (1968) Anorexia nervosa—clinical features and long term follow-up. *J. Chronic Dis.*, **21**, 361–367

STEINHAUSEN, H.-C. and GLANVILLE, K. (1983) Follow-up studies of anorexia nervosa: a review of research findings. *Psychol. Med.*, **13**, 239–249

SWIFT, W. J. (1982) The long-term outcome of early onset anorexia nervosa. *J. Am. Acad. Child Psychiatry*, **21**, 38–46

THEANDER, S. (1970) Anorexia nervosa: a psychiatric investigation of 94 female patients. *Acta Psychiatr. Scand.*, suppl. 214

TOLSTRUP, K., BRINCH, M., ISAGER, T., NIELSEN, S., NYSTRUP, J., SEVERIN, B. and OLESEN, N. S. (1985) Long-term outcome of 151 cases of anorexia nervosa. *Acta Psychiatr. Scand.*, **71**, 708–787

WILLIAMS, E. (1958) Anorexia nervosa: a somatic disorder. *Br. Med. J.*, ii, 190–195

Chapter 18

Bulimia nervosa

Ever since Gull's presentation of the history of Miss A (Gull, 1874), it has been recognized that there are some cases of anorexia nervosa in which the appetite will at times be voracious, or irrespective of hunger, large amounts of food will be consumed within a short time. Bulimia, the term coined to describe such behaviour has acquired two meanings. The first, and original, usage refers to a symptom. Anorectics have, for example, been classified on the basis of whether or not overeating ever occurs. More recently, bulimia has been employed to describe a syndrome, of which binging is only one component. It is this syndrome to which the name bulimia nervosa has been applied. Alternative terms include bulimarexia, the abnormal weight control syndrome, the dietary chaos syndrome, the bulimia syndrome, and the bulimic variant of anorexia nervosa.

Clinical features

Bulimia nervosa was first described and named as such by Russell (1979), who regarded the disorder as a variant of anorexia nervosa. His diagnostic criteria were twofold. First, there was an irresistible urge to overeat, followed by self-induced vomiting, purging, or both. The second feature was a morbid fear of becoming fat. Only two of 30 patients, whose ages at the onset of bulimia ranged from 15 to 37 years, were males. Seventeen (57%) patients had a previous history of unequivocal anorexia nervosa, and a further seven (23%) had experienced milder forms of the illness. The prognosis appeared poor.

Since the original account a number of further descriptions have appeared. The typical case of bulimia nervosa is a female in her early twenties. She will be more sexually active than those with anorexia nervosa, and is more likely to be married and have children. Her family will be in the upper or middle social classes, and the patient will have been well-educated or still a student. Her weight is likely to be normal, but there may be some menstrual disturbances. There is some controversy over the coexistence of psychiatric symptoms, and the significance of a history of anorexia nervosa in the past.

The major clinical feature of bulimia nervosa is the binging. This differs from self-indulgent gluttony as the patient is aware that her behaviour is abnormal and cannot desist even if she does not feel hungry. Furthermore, the binge is often carried out in secret, and follows an unwelcome event or feelings of anxiety, depression, boredom, or loneliness. The gorging will continue until either the patient or her supply of food is exhausted, or it is interrupted by pain, sleep, vomiting, or the arrival of company. Instead of feeling well-satisfied, the patient will be guilty, unhappy, and ashamed. Some may feel drowsy afterwards, and there are descriptions of binging occurring in an altered state of consciousness when everything seems hazy. Hence estimates of the food consumed are not always reliable. Claims of as much as 55 000 calories per binge have been made, and because of the expense involved some bulimics are driven to steal money or food, or raid rubbish-bins. The food eaten is not normally part of the patient's diet, and frequently consists of sweet or salty carbohydrates of a texture which makes them easy to swallow. If vomiting is intended, large volumes of fluid may be taken as well. Most bulimics binge at least once a day, usually in the evening, and some will vomit or purge even after a normal meal. Many cases report periods of controlled eating in between spells of binging behaviour. However, even at such times eating habits may still be abnormal. Some patients will virtually starve, others will spit out food, and some may regurgitate and ruminate.

About 75% of bulimics rid themselves of food by vomiting. This is commonly achieved by inserting a finger into the throat, but some patients acquire the art of vomiting at will, or by gentle pressure on the abdomen. Purgation appears to be less common, and occurs in about one-half of the cases. Vomiting and purging are usually described as commencing at around one year after the onset of binging, but in a minority may begin concurrently or earlier. Fairburn and Cooper (1984a) compared laxative abusers with those who vomited. The former tended to be older and to have longer histories, but to binge less frequently and be more willing to seek help.

By definition, bulimics have a fear of becoming obese, but only a few are in fact overweight; most have weights within the expected range for their sex, age and height. The weight is usually stable, but in some instances may show marked fluctuations. Amenorrhoea is uncommon in bulimia nervosa, being present in only about one-fifth of cases. Where menstruation does take place it is often irregular, unless the woman is taking an oral contraceptive.

Russell (1979) found that the majority of his patients were distressed by their behaviour, and complaints of depression were common. Eleven cases had made at least one suicide attempt, one successfully. Other studies have confirmed the high prevalence of depression, and Johnson et al. (1982) found that 5% of their 316 cases had seriously considered suicide. Drug or alcohol abuse, and self-mutilation have also been reported (Mitchell and Pyle, 1982; Mitchell et al., 1986). Fairburn and Cooper (1984a) stated that 80% of the bulimics they had investigated could be regarded as psychiatric cases independently of their bulimia. By contrast, Johnson et al. (1982) noted that psychiatric symptoms were less common in bulimia nervosa than in anorexia nervosa, anxiety neurosis, and depressive neurosis.

Eighty per cent of Russell's cases had a history of anorexia nervosa in the past and he regarded bulimia as being a form of this disorder. Other workers have found lower incidences, and Johnson et al. (1982) reported that only 5% of their patients had suffered from anorexia in the past. As has been discussed by Fairburn and Cooper (1984b), some doctors refuse to make the diagnosis of bulimia nervosa if there is a present or previous history of anorectic symptoms. They found it difficult to justify this view as they failed to demonstrate any difference between bulimics with a history of anorexia nervosa, and those without. Lacey (1982) has studied the characteristics of young people of normal weight who have episodes of bulimia followed by vomiting or purgation, but who have never shown any of the typical features of anorexia nervosa. He describes their disorder as the 'bulimic syndrome', and argued that it was more akin to obesity than to anorexia nervosa.

Epidemiology

Russell (1979) took over 6 years to collect his 30 cases. It is now clear that this gives a misleading impression of a low prevalence of bulimia nervosa in the general population; however, it reflects accurately the reluctance of bulimics to seek medical help. While developing and assessing a questionnaire to detect binge-eating, Hawkins and Clement (1980) found that over three-quarters of female psychology students had indulged in binging, as had almost one-half of the male students. Only about 2% of the students, however, had induced vomiting and all these were female. Stangler and Printz (1980) reported on the psychiatric diagnoses of 500 consecutive attenders at a psychiatric clinic for students of the University of Washington. Seventeen females and two males fulfilled their diagnostic criteria for bulimia nervosa. These represented 3.8% of the total sample, and approximately 1.6% of the annual attenders.

Halmi, Falk and Schwartz (1981) conducted a questionnaire survey of 539 summer session students of the State University of New York. Of the 355 respondents, 13% had all the major symptoms of bulimia nervosa. The majority of bulimics were female (87%) and 19% of the female students had bulimia nervosa. A similar study was carried out at the University of Leicester by Clarke and Palmer (1983), although eating pathology was assessed using a questionnaire more relevant to anorexia nervosa. Of the 156 female students who returned the questionnaire, 72 (46%) admitted to having at some time binged and felt unable to stop. The incidences of deliberate vomiting and laxative abuse were, however, considerably lower.

Johnson et al. (1982) sent out questionnaires to 454 women who had written for information on bulimia after reading various articles by the authors, and obtained 316 cases of bulimia nervosa. Using a similar sampling technique, namely a notice in a popular women's magazine, Fairburn and Cooper (1982) identified 499 cases of bulimia nervosa after receiving adequate responses to 669 questionnaires. In order to obtain a sample which was not self-selected the authors carried out a further survey among 369 consecutive attenders at a family planning clinic (Cooper and Fairburn, 1983). Over one-fifth of the women admitted to binging, but only 1.9% of the subjects could be regarded as having bulimia nervosa. Fairburn and Cooper (1984a) have also used a television programme to publicize bulimia; following this they were able to detect a further 579 cases.

Healy, Conroy and Walsh (1985) have recently suggested that studies based on the response to questionnaires may have given too high an estimate of the prevalence both of binging and bulimia nervosa. At first sight their questionnaire revealed that out of over 1000 students, 17.7% of males and 37% of females binged. However, their responses to cross-check questions reduced the prevalence figures to 1.1% and 10.8% respectively. Analysis of the answers to items concerning other aspects of bulimia nervosa, and excluding those who binged less than once a week, showed that the diagnosis of bulimia nervosa applied to only 2.8% of the females and none of the males.

Aetiology

The aetiology of bulimia nervosa is as obscure as that of anorexia nervosa, but as with the latter disorder, the majority opinion is that it originates from psychological stress. The symptom of bulimia has, however, been observed in a number of physical disorders, including obesity (Stunkard, 1961; Gormally et al., 1982). Kirschbaum

(1951) reviewed the literature and mentioned a number of neurological conditions in which compulsive overeating had been described. These included intracranial tumours or trauma, ictal-related phenomena, senile and presenile dementia, and encephalitis.

Critchley (1962) described the hypothalamic, or Kleine–Levin syndrome, consisting of periods of uncontrollable appetite and sleep, and in some cases increased sexual arousal. Reeves and Plum (1969) reported a young woman who changed markedly in appearance, behaviour, and endocrine function as the result of a small hamartoma which destroyed her ventromedial hypothalamus. In addition to a voracious appetite, she had irrational outbursts of anger and aggression, and showed evidence of dementia. Whittier (1976) has drawn attention to the occurrence of bulimia in some cases of Huntington's chorea, and Rosenburg, Herishanu and Beilin (1977) reported five cases of Parkinson's disease who had bulimia which responded to treatment with L-dopa and a decarboxylase inhibitor. Finally, Remick, Jones and Campos (1980) described bulimia as a postictal event in three patients, one of whom was a schizophrenic receiving ECT.

Although most patients with bulimia nervosa do not have any evidence of organic brain disease there are exceptions. For example, Lacey (1982) found that in some of his cases of the bulimic syndrome the disorder had been ushered in by epileptic seizures or 'absences' beginning in puberty. Others have observed that the EEG may be abnormal in some patients who present with compulsive overeating (Johnson, Stuckey and Mitchell, 1983).

As already mentioned a number of those suffering from bulimia nervosa complain of depression and may exhibit exaggerated guilt and self-destructive behaviour. This and the fact that overeating may alternate with periods of starvation have led some to postulate a relationship between bulimia nervosa and manic depressive disorders.

Those who regularly treat anorectics may encounter what is thought to be iatrogenic bulimia nervosa. Dally and Sargant (1966) observed that compulsive overeating, associated in some with food stealing, was not uncommon among their chlorpromazine-treated anorectics, and Crisp (1965) noted that at follow-up two out of 21 patients treated with bed rest and chlorpromazine were vomiting as well as overeating. We employed smaller dosages of chlorpromazine, and found a lower incidence of bulimia after treatment.

Behaviour therapy may also be followed by bulimia nervosa. Of the 27 cases followed-up by Pertschuk (1977), 10 developed bulimia for the first time and most of these indulged in self-induced vomiting. By contrast, none of the patients on whom Bhanji and Thompson (1974) were able to obtain information were overeating. This contrary finding could have been due to considerable differences in follow-up methods, or in the treatment applied. Pertschuk rewarded weight gain, whereas the patients described by Bhanji and Thompson were among the few in which behaviour therapy was directed towards eating normal meals within a reasonable time. However, in view of the natural history of the disorder, particularly as described originally by Russell (1979), it seems likely that bulimia may arise regardless of any treatment received for previous anorexia nervosa.

Medical complications

The major physical complaints, other than menstrual problems and those directly due to binging, are tiredness, abdominal discomfort, dry skin, and dry or brittle hair

(Johnson et al., 1982). On occasions, however, bulimics may present themselves as medical emergencies. One of our cases attended the hospital accident and emergency department in a state of considerable physical distress following an unusually large binge, and Crisp (1977) has given a graphic account of bulimia presenting as semi-stupor associated with pyrexia.

So far as the physical concomitants and complications of bulimia nervosa are concerned, those due to starvation or gross weight loss do not occur. However, bulimics are at considerable risk of complications due to electrolyte disturbance, and those due to overdistension of the stomach and repeated vomiting. These have already been discussed in connection with anorectics who induce vomiting or purge themselves.

Medical management

In contrast to anorexia nervosa, there is no established tradition of medical management of bulimic patients as an alternative to psychiatric treatment. Drug therapy has been used, but there are relatively few published reports, the number of patients described is often small, and the response variable. Carbamazepine (Kaplan et al., 1983), antidepressants (Johnson, Stuckey and Mitchell, 1983) and lithium (Hsu, 1984) have been prescribed on the basis of a possible relationship between bulimia nervosa and the affective disorders. Similarly, anticonvulsants have been employed in view of the not infrequent finding of EEG abnormalities in compulsive overeating (Johnson, Stuckey and Mitchell, 1983). Finally, there is some evidence that methyl-amphetamine may suppress bulimic symptoms (Ong, Checkley and Russell, 1983). A pharmacological approach to the treatment of bulimia nervosa may therefore be worthy of further exploration.

Summary

There is some controversy as to whether bulimia nervosa is a variant of anorexia nervosa or is a disorder in its own right. Epidemiological studies suggest that it may be more common than anorexia nervosa. However, as bulimia nervosa is compatible with relatively normal health, patients are less likely to seek medical attention and may not do so unless complications arise. There is no firmly established form of treatment, but in some cases drug therapy may be beneficial.

References

BHANJI, S. and THOMPSON, J. (1974) Operant conditioning in the treatment of anorexia nervosa: a review and retrospective study of 11 cases. *Br. J. Psychiatry*, **124**, 166–172

CLARKE, M. C. and PALMER, R. L. (1983) Eating attitudes and neurotic symptoms in university students. *Br. J. Psychiatry*, **142**, 299–304

COOPER, P. J. and FAIRBURN, C. G. (1983) Binge-eating and self-induced vomiting in the community. *Br. J. Psychiatry*, **142**, 139–144

CRISP, A. H. (1965) Some aspects of the evolution and follow-up of anorexia nervosa. *Proc. R. Soc. Med.*, **58**, 814–820

CRISP, A. H. (1977) The differential diagnosis of anorexia nervosa. *Proc. R. Soc. Med.*, **70**, 686–690

CRITCHLEY, M. (1962) Periodic hypersomnia and megaphagia in adolescent males. *Brain*, **85**, 627–656

DALLY, P. and SARGANT, W. (1966) Treatment and outcome of anorexia nervosa. *Br. Med. J.*, ii, 793–795

FAIRBURN, C. G. and COOPER, P. J. (1982) Self-induced vomiting and bulimia nervosa: an undetected problem. *Br. Med. J.*, **284**, 1153–1155

FAIRBURN, C. G. and COOPER, P. J. (1984a) Binge-eating, self-induced vomiting and laxative abuse: a community study. *Psychol. Med.*, **14**, 401–410

FAIRBURN, C. G. and COOPER, P. J. (1984b) The clinical features of bulimia nervosa. *Br. J. Psychiatry*, **144**, 238–246

GORMALLY, J., BLACK, S., DASTON, S. and RARDIN, D. (1982) The assessment of binge eating severity among obese persons. *Addict. Behav.*, **7**, 47–55

GULL, W. W. (1874) Anorexia nervosa (apepsia hysterica, anorexia hysterica). *Trans. Clin. Soc. Lond.*, **7**, 22–28

HALMI, K. A., FALK, J. R. and SCHWARTZ, E. (1981) Binge-eating and vomiting: a survey of a college population. *Psychol. Med.*, **11**, 697–706

HAWKINS, R. C. and CLEMENT, P. F. (1980) Development and construct validation of a self-rated measure of binge eating tendencies. *Addict. Behav.*, **5**, 219–226

HEALY, K., CONROY, R. M. and WALSH, N. (1985) The prevalence of binge-eating and bulimia in 1063 college students. *J. Psychiatr. Res.*, **19**, 161–166

HSU, L. K. G. (1984) Treatment of bulimia with lithium. *Am. J. Psychiatry*, **141**, 1260–1262

JOHNSON, C., STUCKEY, M. and MITCHELL, J. (1983) Psychopharmacological treatment of anorexia nervosa and bulimia. *J. Nerv. Ment. Dis.*, **171**, 524–534

JOHNSON, C. L., STUCKEY, C. L., LEWIS, L. D. and SCHWARTZ, D. M. (1982) Bulimia: a descriptive survey of 316 cases. *Int. J. Eating Disorders*, **2**, 3–16

KAPLAN, A. S., GARFINKEL, P. E., DARBY, P. L. and GARNER, D. M. (1983) Carbamazepine in the treatment of bulimia. *Am. J. Psychiatry*, **140**, 1225–1226

KIRSCHBAUM, W. R. (1951) Excessive hunger as a symptom of cerebral origin. *J. Nerv. Ment. Dis.*, **113**, 95–114

LACEY, J. H. (1982) The bulimic syndrome at normal body weight: reflections on pathogenesis and clinical features. *Int. J. Eating Disorders*, **2**, 59–66

MITCHELL, J. E., HATSUKAMI, D., PYLE, R. L. and ECKERT, E. D. (1986) The bulimia syndrome: course of the illness and associated problems. *Compr. Psychiatry*, **27**, 165–170

MITCHELL, J. E. and PYLE, R. L. (1982) The bulimic syndrome in normal weight individuals: a review. *Int. J. Eating Disorders*, **1**, 61–73

ONG, Y. L., CHECKLEY, S. A. and RUSSELL, G. F. M. (1983) Suppression of bulimic symptoms with methylamphetamine. *Br. J. Psychiatry*, **143**, 288–293

PERTSCHUK, M. J. (1977) Behaviour therapy: extended follow-up. In *Anorexia Nervosa*, edited by R. A. Vigersky, pp. 305–313. New York: Raven Press

REEVES, A. G. and PLUM, F. (1969) Hyperphagia, rage, and dementia accompanying a ventromedial hypothalamic neoplasm. *Arch. Neurol.*, **20**, 616–623

REMICK, R. A., JONES, M. W. and CAMPOS, P. E. (1980) Post ictal bulimia. *J. Clin. Psychiatry*, **41**, 256

ROSENBERG, P., HERISHANU, Y. and BEILIN, B. (1977) Increased appetite (bulimia) in Parkinson's disease. *J. Am. Geriatr. Soc.*, **25**, 277–278

RUSSELL, G. (1979) Bulimia nervosa: an ominous variant of anorexia nervosa. *Psychol. Med.*, **4**, 429–448

STANGLER, R. S. and PRINTZ, A. M. (1980) DSM-III: psychiatric diagnosis in a university population. *Am. J. Psychiatry*, **137**, 937–940

STUNKARD, A. (1961) Hunger and satiety. *Am. J. Psychiatry*, **118**, 212–217

WHITTIER, J. R. (1976) Asphyxiation, bulimia, and insulin levels in Huntington disease (chorea). *J. Am. Med. Assoc.*, **235**, 1423–1424

Appendix

Normal values

This table is based on the normal ranges used by our laboratories. Multiply value in SI units by factor to convert to other units.

Estimation	SI units	Factor	Other units
Haematology			
Haemoglobin	1.86–2.48 mmol/l	6.5	12–16 g/100 ml
MCV	75–95 fl	1	75–95 cμ
White cell count	4–11 × 10^9/l	1000	4000–11 000/μl
Platelets	150–400 × 10^9/l	1000	150 000–400 000/μl
Serum biochemistry			
Albumin	32–50 g/l	0.1	3.2–5.0 g/100 ml
Alanine aminotransferase	5–50 IU/l	—	—
Alkaline phosphatase	25–85 U/l	—	—
Aspartate aminotransferase	0–25 IU/l	—	—
Bicarbonate	22–30 mmol/l	1	22–30 mEq/l
Calcium (total)	2.2–2.62 mmol/l	4	8.8–10.5 mg/100 ml
Calcium (ionized)	1.07–1.27 mmol/l	4	4.3–5.1 mg/100 ml
Carotene	0.9–3.6 μmol/l	56	50–200 μg/100 ml
Chloride	96–106 mmol/l	1	96–106 mEq/l
Cholesterol	3.7–6.9 mmol/l	39	145–270 mg/100 ml
Glucose (fasting)	4.2–6.5 mmol/l	18	76–117 mg/100 ml
Growth hormone (fasting)	< 20 mu/l	0.5	< 10 ng/ml
Magnesium	0.7–1.0 mmol/l	2.4	1.7–2.4 mg/100 ml
Phosphate	0.8–1.45 mmol/l	3.1	2.5–4.5 mg/100 ml
Potassium	3.5–5.5 mmol/l	1	3.5–5.5 mEq/l
Prolactin	0–400 mu/l	—	—
Sodium	132–144 mmol/l	1	132–144 mEq/l
Thyroxine (T4)	58–170 nmol/l	0.08	4.6–13.6 μg/100 ml
Tri-iodothyronine (T3)	1.2–2.8 nmol/l	65	78–182 ng/100 ml
TSH	< 5 mu/l	—	—
Urea	2.5–6.6 mmol/l	6	15–40 mg/100 ml
Zinc	11–19 μmol/l	6.4	70–122 μg/100 ml

Index

Abdominal pain, 24, 34, 46, 49, 50, 52, 130
Acanthocytes, 56, 58
Acetylcholine, 11
Achalasia, *see* Oesophagus
Achilles reflex half-relaxation time, 75
Acrocyanosis, *see* Skin
Acrodermatitis enteropathica, 96, 97
ACTH, inappropriate secretion of, 76, 77
Addison's disease, 28
Adrenal glands, dysfunction of, 76–78
Adrenaline, serum levels of, 11
Aetiology, 7–12
  hypothalamic dysfunction, 9–10, 12
  psychological theories, 7–8
  somatic theories, 8–12
Age of onset, 16, 19, 22–23, 51
Alanine aminotransferase (ALAT), serum levels of, 51
Albumin, serum levels of, 27, 41, 51, 57, 68
Alcohol abuse, 18
Aldosteronism, secondary, 65, 67, 78
Alkaline phosphatase, serum levels of, 51, 67–68
Alkalosis
  hypochloraemic, 65
  hypokalaemic, 41, 47, 63, 65, 66
  metabolic, 39, 66, 78
  respiratory, 66
Amenorrhoea, 18, 24, 128
  primary, 18, 24
  secondary, 12, 15, 18, 24
  and weight, 10, 18, 71
Amino acids, deficiency of, 92, 96
para-Aminohippuric acid clearance, 64
Amitriptyline, 108
Amylase, serum and urine levels of, 52
Anaemia, 32, 55–56, 57, 67
Anorexia, 17
Anorexigenic peptide, 12
Anticonvulsants, *see* individual drugs
Antidepressants
  monoamine oxidase inhibitors, 108
  monoamine reuptake inhibitors, 108
  see also individual drugs
Appetite, *see* Anorexia, Binging, Carbohydrates
Aspartate aminotransferase (ASAT), serum levels of, 25, 51
Astrocytoma, hypothalamic, 9
  histochemistry of, 11
  and hypoglycaemia, 79

Behaviour therapy, 102–104
Benzodiazepines, 107
Beri-beri, 93

Bethanicol, 110
Bicarbonate, serum levels of, 66
Bilirubin, serum levels of, 51
Binging, 24, 34
  see also Bulimia
Birth complications
  and aetiology, 37, 40
  and prognosis, 123
Bleeding time, 58
Blindness, 16
Blood pressure, *see* Hypotension
Blood volume, reduced, 28, 64, 65
Body image disturbance, 7, 16, 24
Bombesin, 12
Bone marrow, 25, 57–58
Bradycardia, 3, 24, 25, 27, 28, 29, 35, 74
Brain damage, in infancy, 37, 40
Breasts, size of, 18, 24, 25
Bromocriptine, 106
Bromsulphthalein excretion test, 51
Bulimia, 5, 11, 17, 24, 37
  see also Binging
Bulimia nervosa
  aetiology of, 129–130
  amenorrhoea in, 127, 128
  anorexia nervosa and, 127, 128
  binging in, 127–128
  cerebral atrophy in, 41
  plasma cortisol levels in, 76
  depression in, 128
  diagnostic criteria for, 127
  epidemiology of, 127, 129
  hypercarotenaemia in, 89, 90
  iatrogenic, 119, 130
  myopathy in, 42
  prognosis of, 127
  suicide in, 128
  treatment of, 131
  vomiting in, 127, 128
  weight in, 127, 128

Calcium
  dietary intake of, 68
  serum levels of, 25, 67–68
  urinary excretion of, 65
Calf blood flow, 27
Carbamazepine, 109, 131
Carbohydrates
  avoidance of, 17, 22, 23–24
  metabolism of, 78–82
Cardiothoracic ratio, 28–29
Carotene
  bulimia nervosa and, 89

Carotene—*cont.*
   dietary intake of, 88–89
   metabolism of, 89, 95
   pigmentation due to, 18, 24, 25, 88
   serum levels of, 88–90
   vomiting and purging and, 89–90
   zinc deficiency and, 89
Cell-mediated immunity, 60
Cerebellar atrophy, 39, 40
Cerebral atrophy, 39–41
Chest radiography, 25, 27–29, 34–35
Chloride, serum levels of, 38
Chlorpromazine, 107, 113–120
   side-effects of, 37, 107, 113, 114, 118
Cholecystokinin, 12
Cholesterol
   binging and, 87
   dietary intake of, 86–87
   metabolism of, 87
   serum levels of, 86, 87
   see also Hypercholesterolaemia
Circulation, peripheral, 27, 78
   see also Acrocyanosis, Calf blood flow
Classification
   bulimic/non-bulimic, 5, 17, 87
   dieters/vomiters and purgers, 5, 24, 39, 87, 89
   primary/secondary, 5
Clomiphene, 72
Clomipramine, 108
Clotting time, 96
Cognitive deficits, 37, 39–40
Cold, sensitivity to, 24, 74
Colitis, necrotizing, 50
Colon
   dilatation of, 50, 51
   motility of, 51
   obstruction of, 50
   perforation of, 50
   ptosis of, 48
   purgative abuse and, 51
Common peroneal nerve, damage to, 43
Constipation, 19, 24, 46, 50, 52, 74
Copper
   deficiency of, 97
   treatment with, 97
Corticotrophin-releasing hormone (CRH), 76–77
Cortisol, 75, 76–77
Craniopharyngioma, 9, 10
Creatine (phospho)kinase, serum levels of, 41, 42
Creatinine
   clearance, 64, 66
   serum levels of, 25, 63, 64
   urine levels of, 64
Crown–Crisp Experimental Index, 18
Cushing's syndrome, 77–78
Cyproheptadine, 108

Defence mechanisms, 101
Definitions, *see* Diagnostic criteria
Dehydration, 27, 39, 55, 63
Delayed hypersensitivity, 60
Dental erosion, 46–47

Depression, 11, 19, 24, 37, 71, 76, 117
Dermatitis artefacta, 19, 23
Development, retardation of, 12, 92–93
Dexamethasone suppression test, 76, 77
Diabetes insipidus, partial, 64, 71
Diabetes mellitus, 17, 23
Diagnostic criteria, 4–5, 15–16, 22
Diarrhoea, 46
Dietary knowledge, 92
Dieting, 16
Diuretics
   abuse of, 17, 24, 63
   and magnesium deficiency, 67
   and potassium deficiency, 65
Domperidone, 110
L-Dopa, 10, 106, 130
Dopamine
   activity in hypothalamus, 10, 76
   antagonists, 10, 73
   metabolism of, 11
   serum levels of, 11
Down's syndrome, 9, 15
Drowsiness, as a side-effect, 118
Drug abuse, 18
Duodenum
   motility of, 48
   obstruction of, 50, 52
   ulceration of, 23, 48
Duration of illness, 23, 113
   and bone changes, 68
   and breast size, 18, 24–25
   effect on the electroencephalograph, 38, 39
   effect on prognosis, 119
   effect on weight gain, 116
   and heart size, 28
   and kidney function, 63
Dysphagia, 42, 46
Dyspnoea, 24, 27, 31

Eating habits, 16, 92
   see also Carbohydrates
Early fasters, 1–2
   Balan, Jane, 1
   Fancher, Mary (Mollie), 1
   Jacob, Sarah, 1–2
   Mary, Queen of Scots, 1
   'miraculous fasters', 1
   Richard II, King of England, 1
Echocardiographic findings, 28, 31
Electrocardiographic findings, 29–30, 31, 41, 65
Electroencephalographic findings, 38–39, 40
   in bulimia nervosa, 130
Electromyographic findings, 41–43
Emaciation, 18, 24, 25, 32
Emetic abuse, 17
   see also Ipecac
Emetine, *see* Ipecac
Emotional stress, antecedent, 2, 4, 7, 16, 18, 24, 71
Emphysema, surgical, 34–35
Epidemiology, of anorexia nervosa
   age, 15, 22

Epidemiology, of anorexia nervosa—*cont.*
  marital status, 22–23
  race, 15
  sex, 15
  social class, 15, 23
Epidemiology, of bulimia nervosa, 127–129
Epilepsy, 23, 37, 38, 130
  iatrogenic, 37, 118
Erythrocyte(s)
  mean corpuscular haemoglobin concentration, 55
  mean corpuscular haemoglobin content, 55
  mean corpuscular volume, 55, 95
  morphology, 50, 56, 95
  sedimentation rate (ESR), 25, 58
  viscosity, 56
  see also Acanthocytes, Haematocrit, Haemoglobin
Examinations, as precipitating stress, 8, 16, 24
Exercise, 2, 16–17
  see also Hyperactivity
Extrapyramidal side-effects, 115, 118

Family stresses
  and aetiology, 7–8, 16, 24
  and prognosis, 123–124
Family therapy, 8, 104
Fasters, early, *see* Early fasters
Fat, loss of, 18, 24, 25, 28, 43, 46, 50, 92
Fatigue, 24, 27, 31
Fatty acids, deficiency of, 96
Fibrinogen, plasma levels of, 58
Flupenthixol, 108
Folic acid, deficiency of, 94–95
Follicle-stimulating hormone (FSH), 72
Freud, Sigmund, 7, 101
Frusemide, 115

Gastric inhibitory polypeptide (GIP), 12
Gastrin, 12
Gastrointestinal radiography, 48, 50, 52
Gastroscopy, 48, 49
Glioma in region of third ventricle, 9
Glomerular filtration rate, 63, 64
Glucagon, 12, 78, 82
Glucose, serum levels of, 12, 78, 79
  see also Hypoglycaemia
Glucose tolerance test, 12, 79, 80, 81, 82
γ-Glutamyltransferase, serum levels of, 51
Gonadal function, 71–73
Granulocytes, *see* Leucocytes
Growth, retardation of, 12, 92–93
Growth hormone, serum levels of
  fasting, 79
  during glucose tolerance test, 79–82
Gull, Sir William, 3, 4
  on aetiology, 3
  cases of Miss A, Miss B, and Miss C, 3
  on diagnosis, 3, 5, 19
  on prognosis, 3, 121
  on treatment, 3, 5

Haematocrit, 55, 57, 63
Haemoglobin, 25, 55–56, 57, 63
  see also Anaemia, Erythrocytes
Haemorrhoids, 46
Hair
  axillary, 18
  in bulimia nervosa, 130
  hirsutism, 23
  lanugo, 18–19, 24, 25
  pubic, 18, 25
Headache, 24, 118
Haloperidol, 114
Heart
  block, 30
  failure, 32, 67, 69
  murmurs, 27
  size, 25, 27–29
  see also Myocardium
Herpes simplex, encephalitis due to, 60
Hirsutism, *see* Hair
Homovanillic acid (HVA)
  cerebrospinal fluid levels of, 11
  urine levels of, 11
5-Hydroxyindoleacetic acid (5HIAA)
  cerebrospinal fluid levels of, 11
  urine levels of, 11
Hyperactivity, 3, 17
  see also Exercise
Hypercarotenaemia, 25, 87–90
  see also Carotene
Hypercholesterolaemia, 86–87
  see also Cholesterol
Hypermagnesaemia, 65
  see also Magnesium
Hyperthyroidism, 74
  see also Thyrotoxicosis
Hypoalbuminaemia, 39
  see also Albumin
Hypocalcaemia, 32, 67–68
  see also Calcium
Hypochloraemia, 65, 66, 78
  see also Chloride
Hypocomplementaemia, 59–60
Hypoglycaemia, 9, 79, 82
  as a side-effect, 37, 118, 119
  see also Glucose
Hypokalaemia, 25, 30, 32, 41, 49, 65, 66, 67, 78
  see also Potassium
Hypomagnesaemia, 67
  see also Magnesium
Hyponatraemia, 65, 66, 67, 78
  see also Sodium
Hypophosphataemia, 69, 106
  see also Phosphate
Hypopituitarism, 4
Hypoproteinaemia, *see* Protein
Hypotension, 24, 25, 27, 30, 31, 35
Hypothalamus
  dysfunction of, 30, 75–76
  tumours of, 8–10, 11, 71
Hypothermia, 2, 3, 25, 38
  see also Thermoregulation

Hypothyroidism, 74, 86
Hypovolaemia, *see* Blood volume

Immunoglobulins, plasma levels of, 59
Infection, risk of, 58–59, 60
Influenza antigens, responses to, 59
Insomnia, 24
Insulin
   hypersensitivity to, 79, 107, 119
   serum levels of, 12, 82
   side-effects of, 37, 113, 118
   treatment with, 106, 113–120
Intelligence, 15, 37, 40
Intestine, small, *see* Small intestine
Intravenous feeding, *see* Parenteral nutrition
Inulin, clearance of, 64, 66
Ipecac abuse
   and cardiomyopathy, 31
   and myopathy, 42–43
Iron
   deficiency of, 56, 94
   serum binding capacity for, 56
   serum levels of, 56
Isocarboxazid, 108

Jejunum, dilatation of, 48

Kidney
   calculi, 65
   function, 63–64, 66
   histology of, 66–67, 78
   plasma flow, 64
   see also Nephropathy
Klinefelter's syndrome, 9
Kwashiorkor, 92, 96

Lactate dehydrogenase (LDH), serum levels of, 51
Lanugo, *see* Hair
Lasegue, Charles, 3–4
   on aetiology, 4
   on prognosis, 4, 121
   on treatment, 4
Lateral hypothalamic syndrome, 9
Laxative abuse, *see* Purgative abuse
Leucocyte(s)
   count, 25, 55, 56–57
   granulocyte adherence, 59
   granulocyte bactericidal activity, 59
   hydrocortisone, response to, 58–59
   leucopenia, 55, 56–57, 58, 59, 118
   lymphocytosis, relative, 55, 57
   mitogenic stimuli, response to, 60
   monocytes, 58
Lipase, serum levels of, 52
beta-Lipoprotein
   and acanthocytosis, 56
   and hypercholesterolaemia, 87
   serum levels of, 56
Liquorice, 41
Lithium, 108–109, 131

Liver
   function tests, 51
   histology, 51
Low T3 syndrome, 74–75
Luteinizing hormone (LH), 71–72

Magnesium
   deficiency of, 67–68
   serum levels of, 29, 67
Male cases of anorexia nervosa, 19
Management
   medical, 105–120
   pharmacotherapy, 106–110
   psychiatric, 101–104
Medulloblastoma of fourth ventricle, 9
Melanosis coli, 51
Melatonin, plasma levels of, 82
Mental handicap, 15, 23
Methylamphetamine, 131
3-Methoxy-4-hydroxyphenylglycol (MHPG), urine levels of, 10, 11
Metaclopramide, 48, 109–110, 115
Midbrain tumours, 8–10
Mineralocorticoid excess, 78
Mitral valve prolapse, 31
Monoamine oxidase, in platelets, 11
Morton, Richard, 1, 2–3
   on aetiology, 2
   cases of Miss Duke and Master Steele, 2–3
Muscle
   histology, 41, 42
   weakness, 29, 41–43, 66, 67, 93, 106
   see also Myopathy
Myocardium
   damage to, 30, 31
   efficiency of, 30–31
Myopathy, 31, 41–42

Naloxone, 110
Nausea, 24, 46, 49
Nephropathy, hypokalaemic, 66–67, 68
Neuroleptics
   treatment with, 107–108, 113–120
   side-effects of, 118
   see also individual drugs
Neuromuscular disorders, 41–43
Neuropathy, 42
Neurophysiology, 10–12, 41–42
Neuropsychology, 37–38, 39–40
Neuroradiology, 39–41
Neurotensin, 12
Nicotinic acid, deficiency of, 94
Nocturia, 24, 41, 63, 65, 66
Noradrenaline
   cerebrospinal fluid levels of, 11
   metabolism of, 10–11
   receptor blockade, 106
   serum levels of, 11
   subcortical activity of, 10
Nutritional knowledge, 92

Obesity
  fear of, 16, 24, 117
  as a precipitant, 16, 17, 34
  after treatment, 119
Oedema, 25, 27, 63, 65, 78, 115, 118
Oesophagus
  achalasia of, 48
  dilatation of, 48
  motility of, 34, 48
  perforation of, 49
Oestradiol, plasma levels of, 72
Oestrogen
  deficiency of, 68, 92
  hypothalamic hypersensitivity to, 106
Older cases of anorexia nervosa, 19, 22
Opioids
  antagonists of, 110
  in cerebrospinal fluid, 11
Oral contraceptives, 24
Orphenadrine, 115
Osteomalacia, 25, 68, 95
Osteopenia, 68
Ovaries
  cysts of, 23, 46, 72
  functioning of, 72

Pancreas
  atrophy of, 52
  inflammation of, 52
Pancreatic polypeptide, 12
Parasuicide, 18
Parathyroid hormone, 68–69
Parenteral (intravenous) nutrition, 105–106
Parotid glands, enlargement of, 47
Patterson–Brown–Kelly syndrome, 56
Pellagra, 38, 94
Pericarditis, 31
Phenelzine, 108
Phenoxybenzamine, 106
Phenylalanine
  blood levels of, 11
  cerebrospinal fluid levels of, 11
Phenytoin, 109
Phosphate, serum levels of, 25, 67–68, 69
Physical illness
  antecedent, 8, 19
  concurrent, 23
Pimozide, 107, 114–120
Pineal gland, 82
Pinealoma, 9, 82
Pituitary fossa, 39
Pizotifen, 109
Plasminogen activator, 58
Platelets, 25, 57
  see also Thrombocytopenia
Pneumomediastinum, 34–35
Pneumonia, 34, 49, 58, 106
Pneumopericardium, 34
Pneumothorax, 34, 106
Positron emission tomographic findings, 41

Potassium
  deficiency of, 41, 66, 67
  serum levels of, 38, 66
  urine levels of, 66
  see also Hypokalaemia
Procyclidine, 115
Progesterone
  plasma levels of, 72
  treatment with, 106
Prognosis, 121–125
  age of onset and, 122
  assessment of, 121–123
  birth complications and, 123
  cognitive deficit and, 37
  family background and, 123–124
  marital status and, 123
  precipitating factors and, 124
  psychopathology and, 124
  religion and, 123
  response to treatment and, 124–125
  sex and, 123
  social class and, 123
  treatment and, 104, 121
  variability of, 121
  vomiting and purging and, 17, 118, 122–123
  weight loss and, 122
Prolactin
  serum levels of, 73
  response to TRH, 73–74
Propranolol, 106
Protein
  catabolism of, 63
  dietary intake of, 92, 96
  plasma levels of, 51, 64
Prothrombin time, 51, 96
Psychoanalysis
  and aetiology, 7
  treatment by, 101, 102
Psychotherapy
  interpretive, 101
  supportive, 102
Pulmonary abscess, 34, 35
Pulse rate, see Bradycardia, Electrocardiographic findings, Tachycardia
Purgative abuse, 5, 17, 24, 41, 46, 52, 113, 127
  effects on colon, 51
  and dehydration, 65
  and magnesium depletion, 67
  and potassium depletion, 65
  and prognosis, 17, 118, 122–123
Purpura, 57, 94, 95
Pyloric obstruction, 48

Rectal prolapse, 46
Red blood cells, see Erythrocytes
Reverse T3 (rT3), 74

Scurvy, 94
Self-mutilation, 18
Serotonin
  antagonists, 108, 109
  metabolism of, 11

Skin
  acrocyanosis, 18, 24, 25
  callosities, 47
  dryness of, 18, 24, 25, 74
  infections, recurrent, 59
  pigmentation of, 18, 24, 25
  rash, as side-effect, 118
  temperature, 2, 27
Small intestine
  motility of, 48, 49
  obstruction of, 69
Sodium
  conservation of, 65, 66
  deficiency of, 66
  serum levels of, 38, 64
Somatomedin, 79, 80
Somatostatin, 12
Stomach
  acidity, 47
  dilatation of, 34, 49–50
  motility of, 48
  rugal hypertrophy of, 48
  rupture of, 49
  ulceration of, 50
Submandibular gland, enlargement of, 47
Submaxillary gland, enlargement of, 47
Sulpiride, 108
Superior mesenteric artery syndrome, 50, 52
Syncope, 30

Tachycardia, 31, 32
Teeth, *see* Dental erosion
Testosterone, serum levels of, 72
delta-Tetrahydrocannabinol, 106
Thermoregulation, 10, 71
Thiamine, deficiency of, 93–94
Thrombocytopenia, 57, 96
Thymulin, 60
Thyroid-stimulating hormone (TSH), 74, 75
Thyrotoxicosis, 17
Thyrotropin-releasing hormone (TRH), 12, 75, 76
  test, 73, 75, 76
Thyroxine (T4)
  metabolism of, 74–75
  serum levels of, 74, 76
Tongue, 46, 93
Transaminases, serum levels of, 51, 106
Tranylcypromine, 108
Tri-iodothyronine (T3), serum levels of, 74
Trimipramine, 108
Tryptophan, blood levels of, 11
L-Tryptophan, 108
Tube feeding, 105
Tuberculosis, 34
Turner's syndrome, 8, 23
Tyrosine, plasma levels of, 11

Ultrasonographic findings
  pancreas, 52
  pelvis, 72
Urea
  renal clearance of, 66
  serum levels of, 25, 63, 66
Uric acid, serum levels of, 42
Urine, impaired concentration by kidney, 64

Vasoactive intestinal polypeptide (VIP), 12
Vasopressin, 64, 66
Vitamin A
  deficiency of, 95
  dietary intake of, 95
  metabolism of, 87, 88, 89
  serum levels of, 88, 89
Vitamin B_{12}
  deficiency of, 94–95
  serum levels of, 95
Vitamin C, deficiency of, 94
Vitamin D
  deficiency of, 67
  dietary intake of, 95
  and nephrocalcinosis, 65
  osteomalacia and, 25, 95
  osteopenia and, 68, 95
  serum levels of, 67, 68, 95
Vitamin deficiency
  diagnosis of anorexia nervosa and, 93
  rarity of, 92
  skin manifestations of, 18
Vitamin E, deficiency of, 95
Vitamin K, deficiency of, 95–96
Vomiting, 24, 46, 49, 50, 52
  self-induced, 5, 17, 24, 31, 34, 37, 41, 46–47, 49, 113, 127, 128, 130, 131

Weight loss, 16–17, 22, 23, 24, 113, 128
Wernicke's encephalopathy, 94
White blood cells, *see* Leucocytes

D-Xylose absorption, 49

Zinc
  acrodermatitis enteropathica and, 96, 97
  carotene metabolism and, 89, 96
  deficiency of, 97
  hair levels of, 96
  hypogeusia and, 96, 97
  neutrophil levels of, 96
  serum levels of, 96–97
  treatment with, 97, 110
  urine levels of, 96